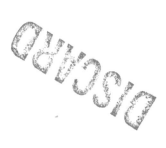

DOWN
SIZE

Foreword by
MEHMET C. OZ, MD

DOWN SIZE

12 Truths for Turning Pants-Splitting Frustration into Pants-Fitting Success

TED SPIKER

HUDSON
STREET
PRESS

HUDSON STREET PRESS
Published by the Penguin Group
Penguin Group (USA) LLC
375 Hudson Street
New York, New York 10014

USA | Canada | UK | Ireland | Australia | New Zealand | India | South Africa | China
penguin.com
A Penguin Random House Company

First published by Hudson Street Press, a member of Penguin Group (USA) LLC.

LIBRARY OF CONGRESS CATALOGING-IN-PUBLICATION DATA
Spiker, Ted.
    Down size : 12 truths for turning pants-splitting frustration into pants-fitting success / Ted Spiker ; foreword by Mehmet C. Oz, MD.
        pages cm
    ISBN 978-1-59463-191-7
1. Spiker, Ted—Health.   2. Weight loss.   3. Overweight persons—United States—Biography.   I. Title.
RM222.2.S678 2014
613.2'5092—dc23
[B]
                2014015115

Printed in the United States of America
10 9 8 7 6 5 4 3 2 1

Set in Janson Text LT Std
Designed by Eve Kirch

To my wife, Liz, for teaching me about
the real meaning of passion . . .

To my boys, Alex and Thad,
for inspiring me every day . . .

Contents

PART 1: Up Size: Getting Stuck

PART 2: Down Size:
Getting Going

PART 3: Your Best Size:
Getting the Body You Want—for Good

Foreword

I've worked with Ted Spiker for a decade. As one of the coauthors of the *YOU: The Owner's Manual* series that Michael Roizen and I created, Ted served as the primary writer of books about dieting, aging, beauty, parenting, and more. His job: make health not only informative but also entertaining. Our mission in those books was to help people learn how the body works and figure out the strategies they can use to live a healthier life. What we found was that people like getting their health information this way—they like to learn, and they like to laugh. (I'd say it's like a spoonful of sugar helping the medicine go down, but nobody needs any more sugar.)

That's a primary reason Ted's book *Down Size* is one that anybody who has struggled with weight can relate to. It's fun. It's real. And it will help you think about the entire issue of being overweight or obese in a way you never have before. Too often, we all may be guilty of simplifying dieting and weight loss as we desperately search for magic bullets that will make fat melt away. But the reality is—and I know this not only from the science perspective, but also from having worked with thousands of people struggling to lose weight—the battle is nuanced. Don't think of weight loss as a series of steps, but more as a set of overlapping circles. You need to know about nutrition and exercise, yes, but you also need to know about psychological aspects such as motivation and connecting with the people around you. And that's what Ted's book is about—finding the twelve truths that will help anyone in their quest for a better, healthier body.

You know what's funny? Even though we've spent hours and hours on the phone together, exchanged countless e-mails, and worked together on hundreds of files, I didn't know much about Ted's personal struggles. (It's not as if he got on the phone every week and confessed, "Hey, Mehmet, that cheesy beef burrito was out of this world.") But I could sense them. Case in point: Ted and I once played one-on-one basketball together. (He details our game starting on page 112.) During the game, he joked around about his physical abilities, and I joked right back—complimenting his use of his ample gluteus maximus to make some room for himself on the court. (That's what we guys do, after all.) Though I'll let him tell you the outcome of our game, I will tell you one thing I noticed about Ted: His determination is a quiet one. That's evidenced by his many attempts to take on challenges in his life—including his attempt to finish an Ironman, an amazing endurance event that's a test of both physical and mental strength. It's that determination that helped him lose the weight he wanted to and it can help you, too.

In *Down Size*, Ted details his story to take you through the arc of weight gain and weight loss, but the book isn't about just him. He also tells the stories of many other people, and gets advice from some of the world's leading experts when it comes to helping people understand how to formulate a plan for getting a healthier body. He doesn't present just one point of view, but many—from a variety of experts, from men and women, from those who have succeeded, and from those still trying their darnedest to lose the weight. What I most like about Ted's truths are that they work together—taking into consideration that people aren't robotic followers of a "do this, do that" mentality but, rather, three-dimensional creatures with back stories, and personal preferences, and obstacles that always seem to get in the way. When you read what Ted says about motivation, you'll not only find tricks that can help spark desire, but you'll also discover that motivation is closely related to other ideas, such as the best way to make goals and the best way to use competition to your advantage. That's the way it works in real life: Everything is connected.

Having operated on thousands of people and having hosted *The Dr. Oz Show*, I've seen what's inside people's chests—literally and metaphorically. And I can tell you that perhaps the greatest challenge we have in health care is this: finding ways to get people from knowledge to action. Nobody knew this better than Ted. Here he was, writing diet books, and he had gained a lot of weight. In fact, the most he ever weighed was when he was in the midst of writing about diets and health. There are, of course, many reasons for that. Maybe it was the stress of deadlines, or the pressure to produce, or the fact that his butt had to be tied to his chair for so long every day, or any other number of factors. But the fact that Ted weighed as much as an offensive lineman while spending so much time with diet information points to the very conflict that so many of us have: Even if you know what to do, that doesn't guarantee that you can do it. So there has to be something that bridges the areas of knowledge and action; that's exactly what many of us in health care are after.

Within the stories in this book, you will find lessons and ideas—ones that you can use, that you should try, and that will work. But take note: There's no single right way. There's your way.

Ted found his way, and he can help you find yours.

—Mehmet C. Oz, MD
New York–Presbyterian/Columbia University heart surgeon
Emmy Award–winning host of *The Dr. Oz Show*

Introduction:
Easier Said Than Done

As I scrolled through the comments on my semester's-end evaluations (the place where students can rate their professors anonymously), I stopped the cursor on one sentence. In its brevity, it whispered among the hundreds of other observations. In its content, it sounded like a stadium full of cowbells, amplifying the angst I feel every burger-loving day. Most students use the rating system to praise or slam the class, the readings, or the instructor, but one person, under the heading "Additional Comments," had noted, "Wear slacks that aren't as baggy."

Though I could debate the appropriateness of an undergraduate chirping about my appearance, I couldn't argue with the comment's simplicity and veracity. *Sure, your class is fine. Your pants? Not so much, big boy.*

I've lived most of my adult life in an XXL body with a shape that's genetically and gender-ly damning: I'm a man with a classic pear shape. I carry my extra weight not in my gut, but in my hips, butt, and thighs. Therefore, pants with an accurate waist size fit too tight from belly button to knee, and pants large enough to scoot over my hips droop from my waist like a turkey's wattle. I have not found an off-the-rack, well-fitted pair of pants since 1989 (probably the same year I last said "belly button"), and if given the choice, especially when on display in front of 275 students, I'll opt for too baggy over too tight. That means I leave the house just about every day with the question that has hung over my head for most of my adult life: Why can't I get the body I want?

As early as I can remember, I have directed too much thought and worry toward food, fat, and body parts that jiggle. I have cringed about my weight, wished for a different shape, and dreamt about substituting the *s* for an *n* in the word *husky*. I have spent decades feeling the way I imagine most people with body issues do: a psychological cocktail of frustration, embarrassment, and middle fingers to the mirror. Anyone who has experienced a demonic relationship with a scale knows too well the inner conflict. On one hip, you have the long-term pursuit of a better body. On the other, you have the short-term pleasure of spicy sausage sandwiches.

The worst part of it? It's not as if I haven't known *what* to do. Besides teaching, I'm a health writer who has written hundreds of thousands of words about weight loss, diets, and fitness. As a former staffer at abs-happy *Men's Health* magazine and coauthor of the YOU: The Owner's Manual series of books by Dr. Mehmet Oz (a New York–Presbyterian/Columbia University heart surgeon and host of *The Dr. Oz Show*) and Dr. Michael Roizen (the chief wellness officer of the Cleveland Clinic), I've spent hours and hours talking with doctors, trainers, and nutritional gurus about eating and exercise. I've interviewed hundreds of leading medical experts from places such as Yale and Harvard, I've examined weight-loss studies, and I've even tried workouts designed for elite athletes.

I also mainline whipped cream.

That's what makes the arena of dieting so maddening. Even people who don't deal with the subject professionally know the *what*. For the most part, we accept the foundational equations of weight loss. Vegetables > fried foods. Exercise > the couch. When eating a scoop of chocolate chips, one should not measure that scoop via dump truck. Most of us also know the übertruth, too: What you eat matters the most.

But the reality is that even if we know what's right, it hasn't worked. Not for me, not for millions.

Why? Because that simple "what you eat" is determined not only by a chart of good foods and bad foods, but also by so many nuances, complexities, emotions, and psychological and lifestyle factors that make it difficult for anyone to lay out the perfect diet that works for everyone. That's why I believe that most eating plans *can* work. And most eating plans *can* fail.

Along with all the people who weigh more than they want or who have shapes they don't like, I have spent way too much time being on diets, thinking about diets, and feeling guilty about going off diets—and repeating the cycle again and again. Many of us desperately try to lose weight, and we pledge that we'll do anything to do so. But something's not working. While the Centers for Disease Control and Prevention reports that nearly 70 percent of American adults are overweight or obese, the weight-loss industry sees more than sixty billion dollars in revenue every year. These are the two key statistics that perfectly summarize the ping-pong nature of our dilemma: Get fat, get stuck, get going, get stuck, get mad, get sad, get a cupcake. Every so often, whether we're inspired by a new year or shamed by a double-chinned Facebook photo, we sink our energies into the sexiest of potential solutions—solutions that can work, should work, and do work. But along the way, we forget the most important part of the weight-loss equation: We're human, and we all have a story.

The short of mine: I'm in my mid-forties, six foot two, and have spent most days unsatisfied with my weight and physique. I've lived most of my recent adult years in the 220- to 250-pound range—that's an overweight-to-obese body mass index of 28–32. I left college at around 180 pounds (a normal BMI of 23) and weighed nearly 280 some fifteen years later (a BMI of 36, which is defined as obese). (Note: BMI is not the only marker for health, and it has its flaws, but it does provide some parallelism for understanding height and weight ratios if you don't know what a six-foot-two man should weigh.) I love to exercise and have completed mud obstacle races and a marathon. I've also won eating contests and broken a bicycle seat. In my job as a writer and professor, I've been immersed in health information, so I know the basic facts, as do most of us. Fact: Obesity is really a proxy for other life-shorteners, because being overweight is associated with high blood pressure, heart disease, diabetes, and so many other health issues. Fact: Losing weight reduces the risk factors for many of these conditions. Fact: Our health care system is under enormous pressure because of obesity-related problems. Fact: Many experts will tell you that a reasonable expectation for weight loss should be one to two pounds a week, though nobody wants to wait that long. Fact: I ate a bowl of Samoa Girl Scout Cookie–flavored ice cream as I wrote those previous four facts.

For my whole life, I've battled to turn an increase in information into a decrease in pants size.

I knew it, but I didn't get it.

Now I do. Down to a satisfying-for-me two-hundred-pound range, I've learned that weight loss and body acceptance are only partially about foods and plans and calories and training. They're about art, science, and soul.

What I've learned is that for any man or woman who wants to lose weight or get healthier or simply learn to accept that his or her body is perfectly imperfect, it comes down to more than grilled chicken salads. Most of us can't just follow a step-by-step eating plan indefinitely and expect lasting results. It comes down to figuring out not the rules, but the truths—the principles that can guide your actions, that can steer you in the right direction, that can bail you out when things go wrong, that can take into consideration that your brain (and not your belly) is the lead character in the dramatic performance that is weight loss. When you figure out the truths, they're the ones that can then sustain you when eight of your fingers are knuckle deep in movie-theater popcorn and the other two are tsk-tsking you *not* to go there.

Though we all know admirable folks who truly can treat food like fuel and not let any baggage influence choices, many of us eat our meals with psychological side dishes—because eating is personal. It's social, it's emotional, it's addictive, it's fun, it's comforting, it's pleasurable, and it involves creating cheese-filled memories with the people we care about.

While it may feel simple to just go on a plan that a doctor, nutritionist, or author recommends, it's always more difficult than we think, because of the factors that influence decision making. This is why I've learned that this whole issue comes down to twelve truths about the body and brain. I don't believe you can merely take one or two pieces of diet advice, follow a meal plan, and lose weight for the long term. That's part of the solution, but so is looking under the hood to find what inspires you, what motivates you, what stresses you, what things in your life influence *your* body shape and size.

In this book, I'll cover my twelve truths that address weight loss holistically, by examining not just nutrition and exercise, but also things like motivation, inspiration, and temptation. It took me some time to figure out the common principles that successful weight losers share. For so long, I (and maybe you) wanted there to be that one answer that would be *it*—the secret that could change my body. After years of experimentation and lots of trial and lots of error, I realized this is how it works: In today's world, the person who wants to lose weight stands in a messy room with a locked door. We all want the master key to unlock the door, because we think that behind it lies the final answer to getting a fitter and healthier body, but our bodies and brains don't work in a one-problem, one-solution system. There is no master key. To be successful, you have to stop expecting one answer. Instead, look around the room: Some answers will be on a shelf, some will be buried in a closet, and some (which you haven't even considered yet) will be right there on the floor in front of you. When you put them together, that's when it clicks. That's when it works. That's when we stop flailing. That's when it makes sense.

Through the stories of others, accounts of my own successes and failures, and the insights of experts who study these issues, I will outline the big-picture truths that help people successfully lose weight. I didn't have a single epiphany regarding these truths, but a series of smaller ones. It took going through these issues myself, not to mention writing and reporting about them, for me to start getting a handle on how the mind and body work together in pursuit of a healthier, better body.

In the end, when I stopped chasing the easy answer, weight loss got easier.

Science serves as the foundation for many of the truths I believe in; well-studied data do point us to what's better for us healthwise. Do the strategies studied work? Yes. But you know what? The most sound studies in the world don't mean squat if you're in the minority, and the studies don't mean squat in isolation—that is, it's never just one thing that will be the answer; you have to have a three-dimensional picture. That's why it's so difficult to determine the factors that work, because in order for science to do its job, it has to use controls that will allow us to see the effect of a single factor. Real life, however, indicates that successful weight loss involves many variables. That's why I put stock into anecdotal evidence—evidence that may have worked for me, for others, and maybe for you, too. Anecdotal evidence doesn't mean one element is *the* answer, only that it could be *an* answer, part of an answer, or could inspire you to think of the answer that will work. Some in the scientific community place lesser value on individuals' stories, because so many uncontrolled factors may contribute to the success or failure of a weight-loss attempt. But there *is* power in stories—sometimes in the literal information, sometimes in the metaphors, and sometimes in the subtle lessons that nobody but you sees.

To me, that's the missing piece in this whole weight-loss puzzle: Can we arm ourselves with proper amounts of information, experimentation, and inspiration so that we—as individuals with our own stories, struggles, histories, genes, and personality traits—figure out what works best for us? Successful dieters create their own programs that are driven by science, lifestyle, and personality.

The truths I've identified don't work alone: Throughout this book, you'll see the comingling of many of them, with one truth including elements of others. For example, the power of social connections to help people through weight-related issues (detailed in chapter 11) is part of virtually every other truth in the book.

Ultimately, I hope these truths help address the main roadblocks we confront when it comes to losing weight—whether it's busting through a frustrating plateau or manufacturing motivation. And I hope they offer hints at solutions for eating well, exercising, and creating the best possible physical and psychological environments for your body. I'm not here to push a certain program (such as All Carbs Are Bad!) or blame others for my problems (wait until you hear what happened to me in PE class). What I want to do is take you through the arc of weight gain and loss; that's why these truths are arranged chronologically, the way many of us experience weight and body issues: from "oh no" to "aha"—that is, from getting stuck, to fixing the problem, to finding lifelong solutions. For me, these truths revolve around all aspects of the quest for your desired body in terms of appearance, health, energy, and performance.

I have a couple of quick notes before I start. First, I tell you my stories and the stories of others as a way to help you think about the struggles and solutions many of us experience. That doesn't mean that every answer that bubbles up is the best one for you. At the root of those stories, though, are the truths that may resonate with your lifestyle. So when I tell you that flipping tractor tires with a group of friends helped me lose weight, that doesn't mean this is *the* program you have to follow. There are greater points to consider—one, I like flipping tires, which is psychologically important; two, flipping tires has some intensity, which is physiologically important; and three, I did it with people I liked, which is motivationally important. *That* can apply to any activity. Second, the weight-loss industry often does too much delineating between male and female audiences. While, yes, it does make sense to address some issues by gender, because of the genetic and psychological differences between us, I don't think that means weight loss needs to be a gender-specific pursuit, especially when it comes to the psychological side. Example: While it's easy to stereotype men as competitive or women as emotional, why can't one gender learn from the other's traditional gender assignments? Why can't a woman want to whoop some butt as a motivational tactic for losing weight? And why can't a man acknowledge that the reason he ODs on cheese curls is because he's upset with what's going on at work or home, or the outcome of a playoff game or *The Bachelor*? Of course they can, and there are plenty of real-life examples of people who don't follow gender norms. So, you may read things that *feel* male or female, but the gender doesn't make a difference. Fact is, some men do yoga, and some women flip tires. I didn't write this exclusively for men or women, and I tried to draw on stories from both genders. And, really, some men could benefit from the lessons we learn from women (and vice versa). My hope is that this book will resonate with anyone who's been so frustrated with a scale that they've felt like drowning their sorrows in their nasty sugar blob of choice. Of course, when it comes to body issues, women historically have had to deal with much more unfair standards and expectations than men. I'm not trying to minimize *that* aspect of body image and weight loss; I just think if we blur the gender lines a bit, we might see answers in places we wouldn't normally look.

Lastly, I don't assume all dieters have the same reasons to want to lose weight. Some want to look better or feel better. Some do it to live longer or get stronger. Some do it because they think they'll be happier. Some do it because they want to have more life adventures. But I do assume that every dieter is pursuing *something*. As for me, my goals are a mixture of the classics. Yes, I'd prefer to have well-fitting pants and to stop looking so hippy. I also want to lose weight to try new experiences and challenges, to play better ball, to run faster, to be the athlete I never was as a kid. (When losing weight in the past, I spent too much time focusing on the number on the scale rather than the experiences and connections that were helping me get there.)

When it comes to weight, I've had some successes, but I've also had plenty of failures. My all-time low came when I reached my all-time high. It was August 2007, and I stepped on the scale for the first time in quite a while. I knew I'd gained some weight, but I'd been wearing blinders when it came to estimating the amount. The needle catapulted to a place it had never been: 279 bleeping pounds. That was 99 pounds heavier than my weight in high school and throughout most of college. My backside had turned into a bounce house.

A week after I weighed myself—and subsequently bought pants in a size that funked me up real good—I had to return to campus to teach my classes for the fall semester. In one of them, Health and Fitness Writing, we'd explore how to report and write about health and medicine. These stories, by nature, can be part informative and part instructive. As a health writer, I'm supposed to not only know what to do, but also at least to be somewhat of a practitioner of the advice I'm reporting and prescribing.

True, I'm no doctor or trainer, but being a health writer and professor whose pants had the waist circumference of a manhole jibed about as well as coffee and mouthwash. It was August in Florida, and a short walk to the classroom across the street meant that I'd be sweating with the ferocity of Class III rapids. The students in that class turned out to be some of the best I've ever taught—some of them now work as fitness writers and editors themselves—but as I stood in front of them talking about the class, trying to cool down, hiding my lumpy frame behind the lectern, I could only imagine what they were thinking of the hypocrisy of it all.

This dude has written diet books?

Closest this guy has been to a push-up is the bra he needs.

Hey, Prof, your ass is a bell curve!

I knew what I was thinking, what I felt, what I needed to do.

It took some time, but I finally learned to build a better body *and* feel satisfied with it, imperfections and all. I've spent most of my life stuck, engaged in a tug-of-war with my desires—wanting a smaller body *and* enjoying bacon burgers. Now I have the truths that helped me balance the competing forces, and I want these truths to do the same for you. Why? Because I believe, from the bottom of my bottom, that every love handle story should have a happy ending.

PART 1

Up Size:
Getting Stuck

Truth: Your "Extra Gland" Is All in Your Head

D raped only in my underwear, I sat on the crinkly white paper for my annual physical. The doctor finished the usual checks of eyes, ears, and throat, and then asked me a question I'm certain no medical school ever encouraged its students to direct to anyone, let alone a fourteen-year-old boy.

"Do you get embarrassed on the beach," he said, "because of your femininely shaped hips and chest?"

"No," I lied, now scarred by another doctor's visit. (When I was eight, my mother asked if my below-the-chest fat rolls could be tumors.)

It turned out the internist was as on target as he was inappropriate. How could you *not* be embarrassed when you were a boy with fatty hips and a rear bumper that could stop small trucks? It's one thing to be heavy or big-boned, or to know you need to lose some weight. But why did I have to be built like a bottle of wine, with a skinny neck and a wide bottom?

The answer, according to this doctor: "You probably have an extra gland."

An extra gland?

With the nonchalance of someone asking for his dressing on the side, he gave me a half-assed (or, in my case, full-assed) explanation. I was a growing young man who had nearsightedness, a mole on my neck, and an extra gland. Looking back, I wish I had asked him if he had a scalpel so he could remove said gland and then shove it right up one of his own.

Long before the doctor articulated it, I knew my body looked different from those of most guys my age. As a kid, I don't think I ever really looked obese, probably because of my bamboo-thin neck and "aristocratic jawline," as it was once described by one of my sister's friends. But everything except my neck, wrists, and ankles always bordered on doughy. I can't remember stewing about what the doctor said, and I would never blame him for why I had such trouble losing weight as an adult. I do, however, remember that moment as the one that defined what I thought about my body: I was the man with the extra gland.

The Pursuit of Perfection:
What You Want Versus What You Have

In a magazine story I wrote about male body image, I admitted that I admired the bodies not only of women, but also of fit men— a fact that I believe stems partly from the incident I've just mentioned. (It's also a fact that some of my male friends found curious.) As someone who's never sported a classically strong male body himself, I've admired other people's bodies—not in a sexual way, but in a complimentary way. I didn't *want* their bodies. I wanted their *bodies*.

I used to observe an older man who was a member of the same gym I belonged to. Having belonged to a top-notch facility for more than a decade, I've seen the full spectrum of gymgoers: fit college kids, former NFL players, Olympians, newbies, grunters, mirror lovers, women with fake boobs, men who chat up women with fake boobs, men with fake tans, those who do more talking than training, beasts (multiple definitions thereof), and "Matchy-Matchy Men" (guys who own enough pairs of sneakers to go with every color combo of their workout wear). For years, I eyed up one man in particular.

He appeared to be in his seventies and usually wore a tank top and tight gym shorts. He stuck out for me not for his style, but for his body. Dude looked lean and strong. If you'd removed his balding, gray-haired head from his body, you'd have thought he was thirty years old. While many of his saggier peers spent their mornings in aqua aerobics classes, this man lifted weights. He ran sprints on the treadmill. He appeared to have zero body fat. If I went to the gym in the morning, I'd see him there. If I went in the afternoon, I'd see him there. And if I spotted him in the hot tub, I'd say to myself, "Why, for the love of all things au gratin, can't I have a body like that?"

I don't think my envy is unusual (though perhaps my confession that I admire the body of a seventy-year-old man is). Anybody who has tried to lose weight has probably fantasized about having someone else's physique. For a man, maybe it's Brad Pitt, David Beckham, or LeBron James. For a woman, maybe it's Halle Berry, Serena Williams, or Kate (Upton, Middleton, your choice). Whatever you like, whatever you want.

I had never thought I'd be holding up a retired man's body as a symbol of bodily ideals, but there was something about the way he carried himself that just oozed of strength. I figured he must have lived his entire life like an athlete. I admired him, yes, but he also pissed me off, because I had spent most of my life looking like his exact opposite: gooey with periods of not-so-gooey.

One day, I asked a colleague who seemed to know everyone at the gym who this guy was. It felt less creepy than actually approaching the man: *Uh, yeah, hi, sir. I really admire the shape and size of your pectoral muscles, especially for a man of your age.* My friend knew him. He was a retired anatomy professor.

Of course he was.

As soon as I heard that, I knew I had to talk to him—to learn more not just about how he did what he did, but also about fat and muscle, and to ask him a selfish question: Was it indeed biologically possible to sport an extra gland?

Every one of us who has struggled with weight has both a physical and psychological foundation for our problem—perhaps that literal extra gland, or a symbolic one that's ingrained in us as we're growing up and that has an effect on how we see and do things as adults. These psychological foundations influence how and why we gain weight, whether we can lose it, and what we think about our bodies. And they influence our perception of reality: of our ideal bodies and of the actual bodies we have to work with. The metaphorical "extra glands" are the physical and psychological foundation that often come from genetics and from the experiences we don't control. For anyone trying to embark on a weight-loss quest, leaving behind your extra glands is part of the answer.

Your physique—for me, redwood-thick butt, lumpy hips, and apparently some kind of a glandular issue—mingles with the psychological structures we build: How does your body, and your perception of your body, influence who you are? I had several experiences that, I suspect, contributed to a vicious cycle in adulthood, a cycle that went something like this:

My body is no good, so I try to make it better.

When I try to make it better, I embark on a new challenge.

After the initial success, I lose momentum, stall in my quest, tell myself that my body is no good, then fall short of my expectations.

Therefore, I must eat cake batter.

There's a fine line between someone's physical and psychological history and using that history as an excuse: The foundation isn't about blame.

Throughout my life, I can count on two or three fingers the number of times I've felt truly satisfied with my body, but I don't believe I have ever blamed anything or anyone for this. I have never "woe is me" wallowed; I've always taken responsibility for what and why I eat. Identifying these influences that may have played a role in your weight issues isn't about making excuses or whining or shifting responsibility to some other force; it's simply about articulating an explanation, teaching yourself how you're formed genetically (this is the body your parents made for you) and environmentally (this is the body your kindergarten classmates told you looked like a zoo animal)—then dumping both down the garbage disposal.

Understanding these two foundations, I think, is the first step toward turning your body in the direction you want—not because of any magical change it creates in your future actions, but because it gives you a chance to outline facts about your past rather than hide them. It's how I knew I needed to understand a little bit more about how I was built.

So I called on the retired anatomy professor.

When David Kaufmann came to my office, he insisted on biking over in a driving rain. He had worked at the university where I worked for close to thirty years without ever having bought a parking sticker, because he cycled to work every day. Kaufmann played football, basketball, and ran track in high school, and he was an early adopter of weight training to improve athletic performance. Today, at age eighty, he still lifts weights, runs, stretches, and competes in statewide master's competitions in the 400-meter run. I wanted to know about fat—how it's stored and why it chooses to lay squatter's rights where it does. He told me what undergrads used to ask him back when he taught about the body.

"Students, usually women, would come in and say, 'I've got a big bust, what can I do? What's wrong?' Or 'I don't have any fat in my chest,' or 'I've got a big rear end,' or 'How do I get rid of fat in my calves?'" Kaufmann said. "They wanted to know a program to change it. But I had to tell them, 'You have a DNA program that says you're going to lay your fat down there.'"

I figured if he had students who asked him about their big busts, I could, too.

I stood up. My body shape, I told him, felt too tinged with female traits. I stored fat in my hips and butt, not my belly.

"That's right," he said.

Aside from the food, I asked, why am I this way? Why do I have to store my fat like this? I was looking for answers at the cellular level; instead, he gave me one at the jovial level.

"It's really from your mom and dad's DNA. Your mom and

dad conceived you, and part of your dad's DNA and part of your mom's DNA came out with a little boy."

He paused.

"Or big boy."

The Physical Foundation of Fat

Though genetics does dictate the location of fat storage, body shape, and so many other factors in how our bodies develop, we also know that genetics is only one pixel in the fat-loss picture. Having spent many years writing about health, working at *Men's Health* magazine, and collaborating for more than a decade with anatomy lover Dr. Mehmet Oz, I've long believed that changing behavior isn't simply about directives: Do this, do that; eat this, drink that; yes to this, no to that. Changing behavior, and bodies, requires some knowledge about what we're doing and why, and how the body works to store and burn fat.

The simple answer is the one we've all been hammered with: Eat too much without burning it off, and your body stores the fat to use as energy in case you ever come across a time when you run out of it. In an ideal situation, you eat the right amount of fuel to keep up with whatever kind of energy you're expending. If one part of the equation is off (ingest too much, burn too little), your body turns into a human pillow.

That's really the simplest equation that most of us need to know as we're figuring out what works best for weight loss. Yet, as is the case with any of our biological processes, the system is way cooler than a plus-minus equation, and it's not quite as simple (as I'll cover in a few chapters). Some years after my chat with David

Kaufmann, I wanted a refresher course on fat, so I walked across the street from my office at the University of Florida to the College of Health and Human Performance to meet Joslyn Ahlgren, PhD, a lecturer who teaches anatomy and physiology, along with courses in exercise physiology, fitness assessment, and exercise prescription.

Ahlgren, never a science or sports person growing up, worked hard in high school to get out of as many science classes as she could; she even had her parents write notes to teachers to get her out of having to dissect worms. Bored with her major in college, and no longer interested in pursuing broadcast journalism, Ahlgren met someone who told her she should try kinesiology. She ended up switching colleges, took an anatomy and physiology course, and fell in love with learning about the body. "It's an infinity worth of information," she said. "It just doesn't stop."

Very early in our conversation I got the impression that all anatomy professors are ass whoopers: Ahlgren has a black belt in karate, teaches weekly spinning classes, does recreational power-lifting, and (with her husband) has turned her garage into a gym/dojo. Even her supermarket trips turn into workouts. "I refuse to go back and forth to my car to carry groceries," she said. "If I can do it in one swoop, I just have too much ego to go back and get another bag. I'll put it on my pinkie and let my blood supply go away." In her field, she has to live this way. She said she'd feel like a hypocrite if she didn't.

In her Applied Anatomy course, Ahlgren uses texts, lectures, and plastic models to teach students about cells, tissues, organs, and systems. The classes, at close to one thousand students per semester, are too large to include "wet" dissections. "You can imagine having eight or nine hundred eyeballs bouncing around the room," she said, not metaphorically. "We start from the individual Legos and then we build a little car, and then we put the car in the city. We start small and get bigger, but it's a lot of 'why': Does the anatomy make sense?"

I don't want fat to make sense, but it does—and not just in the "I like bacon" kind of way. It also makes sense in the biological way.

The basics: Adipose tissue (fat) consists of a number of different kinds of tissue and serves a variety of functions. For example, fat contains white blood cells, so it plays a role in immunity. It also contains adipose cells, called adipocytes, which are the actual fat cells. (At least 90 percent of adipose tissue cells are adipocytes.) These cells hold triglycerides, fatty acids, for later use as energy. That's the main function of fat—energy storage. Fat can also serve a protective mechanism in the body, guarding organs from potential threats. "If you pluck your eyeball out, the whole back of it is a big wad of fat," Ahlgren said. Fat looks exactly the way you'd think it does: It has a yellow-white tint to it because adipose tissue stores carotene, a substance similar to that which makes carrots orange. (Note: The pinkish color you may associate with fat, if you watch reality shows in which subjects get liposuction, results because adipose tissue is highly vascularized, meaning that when those docs suction fat out of the body, they are also pulling out capillary beds and blood.) Fat also is, as you'd expect, lumpy and greasy. Ahlgren said, "It's not any different than if you go to your local meat market and find a piece of chicken with big chunks of fat on it. It's not any different in humans."

In the past ten or fifteen years, fat has become really sexy, Ahlgren said (now metaphorically, I presume). That's because of its role in the endocrine system—that is, how fat and hormones are related and influence the rest of the body. The hormones secreted by adipose tissue *can* damage the body; that's partly what causes some of the health problems associated with obesity. (Some hormones aren't detrimental when secreted in normal amounts. Leptin, for example, helps inhibit appetite, but chronically elevated levels are associated with obesity and inflammatory disease. "Good hormone gone bad," Ahlgren said.)

What's most important may be the location of the fat. If fat is centrally located, around your organs—that's called visceral fat— it's more damaging than if it's below the waistline, which serves as good news for my long-term health, but not so much for my dressing-room experiences.

We all have to have some fat in our bodies to help with energy storage. The problem is when we have too much. To grow fatter in size, we don't increase the number of cells; we increase the size of the cells. All our food—whether it comes in the form of protein, fat, or carbohydrates—gets broken down so the nutrients can be absorbed into our blood and distributed throughout the body to be used for energy to power our organs and systems. (Our brains, for instance, need a lot of energy.) If you eat too much, your body holds it back for when you're not eating, so those nutrients can keep the body working—to give you a slow and steady feed. If you eat too much and don't use the nutrients, your body stores them as fat.

"It's just like hoarding," Ahlgren said. "You collect too much and now you're stuck with it." (Note to self: I need to clean out my back room.)

Inside fat cells, there's a big balloon full of triglycerides; the more of those triglycerides that go into the fat cells, the bigger those cells swell—essentially, the more bloated the fat cells become, the larger the mass of fat becomes. To lose fat, your body would need to start relying on those stored triglycerides for energy somewhere else—say, for organs while you're exercising. That's when fat cells become smaller—and thus the fat mass gets smaller. The two ways to make this happen: Decrease the energy you take in so that your body needs to go to those stores (i.e., reduce your food intake), or increase the rate at which your body needs to burn calories. This can happen with exercise directly or with the addition of muscle mass. Muscle requires a lot of energy to sustain itself, so by adding some muscle mass, you cause your body to pull from those triglycerides to keep those muscles going. That's what increases your metabolic rate; instead of those triglycerides hanging around the cellular couch, getting fat and happy watching Bravo reality shows, they'll burn off when they go feed the muscle. It's a literal burn into oblivion as your body uses those cells for energy.

Before Ahlgren and I ended our conversation, I felt I needed (once and for all) an answer to the anatomical question I'd had ever since my ding-a-ling doctor gave me his diagnosis.

So I told her about my story and asked if it was possible I had an extra gland.

"Noooooooo," she said, with just enough of an elongated *oooo* to make me, finally, do to my childhood demons what I'd never been able to do with processed meats: throw them away.

"That's just insane to me," she continued. "That's just ridiculous. As far as an actual endocrine organ being present that's not normally present, that's complete bunk. That's just ridiculous. It's one thing to make it sound like it's not your fault, right? You don't want to lay that on a kid and be like, 'You just ate too much, you dork, have some responsibility.' That's not the way to approach it. But completely making something up, that's just asinine."

The Psychological Foundation of Fat

These days, the biological truth about why we store fat where we do might not be all that clear. Traditionally, Ahlgren said, science has always thought that butt and leg fat storage was associated with having more of the female hormone estrogen, and fat storage in bellies was associated with having more of the male hormone testosterone. Certainly some women store fat in their bellies, and some men are shaped like me. Some research shows that men with normal levels of testosterone can have a tendency to store fat in the thighs and gut, too. So the answer about the location of fat storage likely includes some combination of both hormonal influences and genetics.

For those of us trying to lose fat, though, that isn't the most vital mystery to figure out. Losing the fat has less to do with hips and bellies and more to do with stuff deep inside our brains. It's also pretty clear that the physical and psychological factors go together like Cap'n and Crunch. You have a body problem, so that influences how you feel about yourself, how others perceive you, how you think others perceive you, how you perform in whatever activity you're doing, and on and on.

Vincent Felitti, MD, started his medical career in the late 1960s, doing infectious disease work. Early on, Felitti was asked to set up a Department of Preventive Medicine, and he began to study health risks and obesity—and the underlying causes for them. He ran a weight-loss program in San Diego that has treated more than thirty thousand people, and because of the counterintuitive experiences he had while running that program, he became the co-principal investigator with Dr. Robert Anda of the Centers for Disease Control and Prevention of the Adverse

Childhood Experiences (ACE) Study, a joint project between the Kaiser Permanente Medical Care Program and the CDC. Since 1995 the study has looked at the childhood experiences of more than seventeen thousand patients. These folks were middle-class, with three-quarters of them college-educated.

Felitti told me the background story of a woman who came to him in 1985 for help with weight loss. She was twenty-eight years old and weighed 408 pounds. Within a year of an intense calorie-restriction regimen, she dropped to 132 pounds. She stayed that way for six weeks. Then, in a matter of just three weeks, she gained 37 pounds.

Felitti asked her, "What's going on?"

"I think I'm sleep-eating," she said. "As a kid, I was a sleep-walker, but I haven't done it since. Now I wake up in the morning and there are boxes and cans open in the kitchen, somebody's been cooking and eating, and I'm the only person there, so it must be me." And yet she didn't remember doing it.

"Why do you think you're doing it now?" Felitti asked.

"I don't know."

"Why now?" he pressed. "Why not last year?"

"I don't know."

Finally, after Felitti's third try, the woman told him about a man at work who'd approached her and said, "Patty, you look pretty good. How about you and me making it every week."

Though it was a pretty flimsy proposition, Felitti said, that statement led to the woman revealing that she had been a victim of repeated sexual assaults by her grandfather. Later, she quickly regained all her weight. Felitti asked her why she wasn't able to keep her weight down.

"The weight was coming off faster than I could handle," she told him. "My wall was crumbling."

That statement, "My wall was crumbling," was an incredibly common explanation for why people in Felitti's obesity program often couldn't sustain weight loss. It didn't matter whether someone wanted to lose fifteen pounds or a hundred and fifty, Felitti said. The processes were the same, but the intensity levels were different. Fat protects not just our organs, but also our social selves, both physically and sexually. "People expect less of you when you are obese. It's an effective way of de-sexing oneself as well as looking more powerful. Think of the expression 'throwing your weight around,'" he said.

What Felitti and his colleagues found through their years of study was that when they looked at people who had gained large amounts of weight, the weight gain was not slow and progressive in the way that most people portray their gains—as in "It just started creeping up and creeping up, and eventually I looked over and I was three hundred pounds." The more than seventy-five studies associated with the ACE Study indicate that the onset of weight gain is typically abrupt, and often associated with some major life event. The study identified adverse childhood experiences, organizing them into several categories, including emotional, physical, and sexual abuse; emotional and physical neglect; a parental separation or divorce; and household alcohol or drug abuse. In one of the studies published in the *American Journal of Preventive Medicine* (a survey of nearly fourteen thousand people), Felitti and his team found a one-and-a-half-fold increase in severe obesity among those who had experienced four of seven categories of traumatic experiences.

"The life events part is largely never recognized, partly because it is often decades back," Felitti said. "Plus, nice people don't talk about these things. My god, surely you don't ask strangers about them. So we have these huge realms of human experience that are closed to awareness because of that. As we began to discover the prevalence, we started asking about life events routinely."

In his small-group obesity work, Felitti would always open the discussion with two questions that usually aren't asked of people who need to drop pounds. The first: "Tell me *why* you think people get fat—not *how*; that's obvious." The answers, he said, were striking: depression, stress, men leave you alone. The second question (which surely few people think about, especially as we live in a society where the opposite question is always the one that's asked): "What are the benefits of being fat?" The answers turned out to be more of the same, indicating that fat has socially protective benefits: "People leave you alone, men won't bother you." Week after week, month after month, Felitti heard the same things.

Though his program began with structures and strategies for eating right, it developed into a plan dealing less with food and more with helping people understand why they'd become overweight—and how fat acted as a coping tool against some kind of trauma. In fact, Felitti even argues that many public health problems are the result of "compensatory behaviors" such as smoking, alcohol abuse, drug use, and overeating, because these behaviors provide temporary relief from emotional problems caused by traumatic experiences. The key to understanding obesity, Felitti said, is to ask, "How old were you when you started putting on weight? Why do you think it was *then*?"

The focus of the ACE Study was centered on determining in a general population the typically unrecognized prevalence of seriously adverse life experiences in childhood—and their long-term ramifications a half century later. Are such experiences meant to explain why all people gain weight? Of course not, because there's a range of experiences and reasons, and there's also a big difference between severe obesity and simply adding a few pounds. Unrelated studies point to other factors. For example, a recent Harvard University study looked at obesity rates among adolescents with lower socio-economic status and those with lower-educated parents. The Harvard researchers cited practical reasons for why this would happen, such as fewer open areas to play in poorer communities, higher expenses associated with youth sports programs, and ease of access to cheaper and less healthy food. And certainly, for many people, the "why" may be a mixture of a lot of factors, be they very practical ones such as financial stressors or the deeper ones brought out in the ACE Study.

Though I had that minor run-in with my doctor, I hadn't given much thought to the serious childhood experiences that could affect people's weight in their adult life. Of course, I thought, moments of abuse, neglect, and violence could have lingering effects, but I was certainly struck by how common Felitti found they occurred. So I asked him if these so-called adverse experiences had to be on the upper end of the definition of traumatic. "The categories were selected solely because of their commonness in the obesity program. Are they the only ones? My god, no, but they clearly were on the serious end of the spectrum."

I remember having a happy childhood, and certainly none of my experiences would be classified as serious or adverse. I did have a couple of moments when doctors called me fat. I did have some bouts of gym class humiliation (stories forthcoming). My father died of cancer when I was four. And my mother—likely because she had already lost her parents by the time she was twenty-one and then lost her husband and was left with three children under the age of six—was overprotective and kept me from trying out for some sports teams. Though I would have avoided these negative experiences given the choice, I can't say that they would be clinically classified as adverse, with the exception of the death of my father. But—and I'm extrapolating here—many of us do take our childhood experiences with us as we grow up, and these shape who we are, what we think, and what we do.

When Felitti integrated questions about people's adverse experiences into medical screening surveys of patients, his colleagues feared that internists would have to start playing psychologist if they dared ask patients things so personal or strayed into seemingly nonmedical issues. What he found was that patients would simply state what had happened to them, without much discussion, though sometimes with tears. Unexpectedly, they found that the simple act of asking and letting the patient talk for a minute or two significantly reduced doctor office visits in the subsequent year.

"I slowly came to realize that what we were doing was similar to a confession in the Catholic Church," Felitti said. "The idea of a confession may meet some basic human need, telling something shameful about yourself to someone who was important to you and who would still accept you as a human being. The fact that this has been used for about 1,600 years suggests it meets some basic need."

Demolishing Demons:
A Change in Perspective

Lynn Ramsey's mother decided she didn't want an overweight child. Petite like Grace Kelly or Audrey Hepburn, Lynn's mother concluded that if you're fat, you have no friends. So when Lynn was a toddler, her mother would pick her up and put her on a scale.

Every night.

When Lynn grew into a teenager, she was five foot four and weighed about 150 pounds, so her mother sent her to Weight Watchers, and paid for Lynn to go to aerobics classes at the YMCA.

"I remember being called sturdy by my mother. No female wants to be called sturdy—and she still does it," Lynn said. "I think she saw a girl in school who was on the heavy side. I don't really know of any other reason what her issue was. Where she did a good job was messing with my mind."

So Lynn fought back: She'd buy cookies at school and hide them from her mom. Though Lynn was athletic, her weight fluctuated throughout her adult life. She maxed out at 189 pounds, dropped to 155, and now holds steady in the 160 range and has run ten marathons. She remembers that when she had morning sickness during her pregnancy, her doctor told her she could eat whatever she wanted as long as she could keep it down. That was the first time she was ever told that.

It took some time to shake off the messages she received as a child—she credits the unconditional support of her husband for being able to do so—and that helped her develop a healthy attitude toward eating and body image. She also knew that as a mom of two teenage daughters, she needed *not* to create body image issues for them. (Lynn lost most of her weight through exercise and eating in moderation, and not by depriving herself of any particular thing; she doesn't believe in trendy programs and made the decision not to obsess over everything she eats or how she looks.)

"I think everyone, especially women, has their own version of that story," Lynn said. "If you ask twenty women, they may all have body image issues and different reasons for them, but they're all pretty much the same."

Lynn did what many have a hard time doing: She changed her perspective. Instead of obsessing about her weight, she viewed weight management as a journey, not as a success-or-failure or start-end proposition. She did it by changing the way she viewed the moments that very strongly colored her past. She didn't let her mother's words or actions create a self-fulfilling prophecy. "I do blame my mother in some ways," she told me, "but if I didn't have her to blame, I'd blame something else."

My "something else" didn't come from inside the home. Nobody in my family made fun of me for my shape; nobody said I needed to do a hundred jumping jacks a day. And I was never told to eat less to shrink my "stomach tumors." My family generally had balanced meals in terms of both nutrition and portions, unless company was coming, at which point my mother would make four times the amount of food we needed.

As I was growing up, my mom was always a normal weight, though she did spend some years as an overweight child. She gained weight starting in second grade, when she attended a new school, one she didn't like. An only child, my mother ate hearty meals most nights, such as roast beef, mashed potatoes, and gravy. At the end of dinner, she and her mother would often sneak into the kitchen and eat the "snivvies," the bits of leftover meat dipped in gravy. My mother's preferred breakfast, if there was any in the fridge, was potato salad, homemade apple pie, and vanilla ice cream. By sixth grade, she had ballooned up to 140 pounds. At the end of the year, during a field day attended by students and parents, she participated in a relay race. When she got stuck in an inner tube, that's when things changed. "That did it for my parents. Shortly after that, they took me to the doctor," she said. Back in the pre-diet-explosion days, the doc prescribed normal foods and reasonable portions, while still allowing her one dessert a week. By the end of the summer—the summer before she changed schools to one she liked—she lost forty pounds. To this day, she still steps on the scale every day, eats small portions, and walks a few miles every day.

My "something else"—the thing that messes up your mind—most likely came in the form of gym class. Despite the reality of my body type and the fact that I moved slower than a parked car, I liked gym. (This you will find surprising in roughly four minutes.) I liked the games and the sports, but dreaded being measured in what felt like some elaborate word problem. *If you put Spiker in yellow polyester gym shorts and expose him to conditions in which he gets smoked by classmates who are actual athletes, how many push-ups can he do?*

Consider the Presidential Physical Fitness Test, the series of exercises that all kids had to do to determine their level of running, jumping, pulling, pushing, and shuffling between two cones. I usually scored okay on sit-ups, as I recall, but bombed on all things running. The only time I ever scored above a 0 on pull-ups was when I jumped up and over the bar to get 1 and then used my momentum to sorta-kinda get 2. I suspect my gym teacher purposely looked away.

Since these tests rolled around only once or twice a year, I could muster the energy to get through them. The bigger problem with gym class, though, was the all-caps MOMENT—the one time when you, because of your physical inferiority, are left standing in front of everyone with your symbolic zipper down. I did not have one MOMENT. I pluralized it.

My Phys. Ed. lowlights:

Moment 1: I earned a D in sixth-grade gym, presumably because I ranked as the second-slowest kid in class. Later, my teacher allowed me to do sit-ups after school to change my grade so that I could make the honor roll. To this day, I'm not sure which felt worse—the D, or showing up after school to crunch my way up a few points.

Moment 2: Immediately after the final cuts of my eighth-grade basketball team, when one of the school's best shooters didn't make the final roster of twelve kids and I did (victory!), a friend told me that the only reason I had made the team was because I was student government president.

Moment 3: When I changed shirts in the high school locker room before gym and one of the rebel kids, who had lost a ton of weight over the previous summer, singsonged behind my back, clearly directing it toward me, "*L-uh-uh-uh-uh-uh-ve haaaan-dles!*"

Moment 4: During our rotation through gymnastics in high school PE, we tried out all the equipment. When I stepped up on the balance beam, I shook like a maraca. As soon as I placed both feet on the beam, the coach (a gentle teddy bear of a man who was a former football player yet never used his football voice until this instant) summoned the entire class: "SPOTTERS! I NEED SPOTTERS HERE! NOOOOOOOW!" I (*cough*) came down with a (*cough*) cold the day we were scheduled (*cough*) to try the vault.

The event I most remember came one time in middle school when we were doing the 600-yard run in the Presidential Physical

Fitness Test. I decided to take on a new strategy that year. During our warm-up lap, I would take it *really* easy. Save it all for the test. I was sure this would allow me finally to finish better than I ever had before.

During the middle of that warm-up lap, when I felt that the coach could clearly see that I was well behind the rest—I'd done it on purpose!—he yelled out, "Last one takes another lap!"

My heart sank. Plan foiled. On my "another lap," I defiantly walked. Not because I couldn't run, but because I was fuming. I didn't understand. Why, when he knew I struggled, did he have to make it harder? Looking back, I assume he was only trying to give me a kick in the butt, inspire me to go faster. But it backfired. I finished my timed test slower than the group, as usual.

I tried so hard to figure out a way to stick with my peers, only to be separated from them once again. I remember boiling with anger and frustration—again to be defined as the boy in the back. I can't help but think that those experiences laid the foundation for my always feeling like the barge in a world of jet skis.

It turned out to be my two-pronged childhood demon: a big behind, and being behind.

My anatomical extra gland didn't turn out to be real, but no matter how my size has fluctuated over the years, I typically think of myself as the guy who is picked last and the guy who finishes last. It's likely why I've longed for redemption as an adult—trying new challenges, like a marathon and muddy obstacle races. And it's likely why, in 2013, thirty years after my doctor asked about my femininely shaped hips, I signed up for an Ironman, considered one of the most grueling endurance events in the world—a 2.4-mile swim, a 112-mile bike ride, and a 26.2-mile run, all to be completed within a seventeen-hour limit. I wanted to remove my mental extra gland: the voice dripping with self-loathing that was the most powerful demon of all.

Truth: Why, Yes, You Can Outsmart the Cheese Dip

f I had an eating résumé, part of it would read like this:

Experience

Taco Hoarder, eleven years old: Ate twelve of the twenty tacos
served at my family dinner, leaving only four for mother
and two sisters. Midmeal nosebleed, presumably caused
by speed of ingestion.

Volume Seeker, late twenties: Wrote story for a magazine
called "Heaping Helpings," about trying to finish the
largest portions of food served in Delaware restaurants.
Successfully finished all but a pasta bowl at Caffé Bel-
lissimo.

Meat Master, early thirties: Finished seventy-six ounces of
steak in a one-on-one contest. Declared winner. Also ate
fries and ice cream during meal.

Some people's eating histories may look like mine, with challenges accepted and two-story helpings demolished. Others may
have different food moments that stand out: memories of a

grandmother's hedonistic Sunday meal, or a Twinkie packed in your lunch every day, or candy bars snuck into the house *because* they were forbidden. For most of us who've dealt with weight issues (except those whose weight was caused by a medical issue), food is our protagonist and our antagonist. The problem and the solution. The pleasure and the pain. We want the chocolate, we eat the chocolate, we love the chocolate, we savor the chocolate, we hate the chocolate.

Considering all the world's books, articles, studies, viewpoints, products, and programs, it's easy to say that lots of people have possible solutions to the obesity problem. But if we had to sum up the root causes of obesity, it would come down to this: Our ancestors didn't have queso dip.

We know the traditional tale of obesity: In primitive times, mankind had to hunt for food. So we chased, killed, and feasted on animals and collected berries and whatever else from the earth didn't make us vomit. We also had to spend days covering lots of ground to hunt for dinner and feed our families, so we were constantly in motion, burning calories in a time when nobody knew or cared what a calorie was or how it worked. Mountains were stair-climbers. Rocks were dumbbells. Drumming and dancing around the campfire was Zumba. Getting chased by a bloody-mouthed lion was level 12.0 on the treadmill.

This all changed when we could manufacture food, when we took desk jobs, when some scientists and marketers thought if you combined words that sounded perfectly natural (*fruity* and *pebbles*), you could make a whole lot of money with a whole lot of sugar and its counterparts. As our activity levels dropped, our food choices soared. Of course, the way we gain and lose weight in terms of calories and nutrition isn't as simple as that (more on that soon). The great psychological force put in play for those of us who've had eating and weight problems—temptation—is one that our ancestors didn't have to deal with, because there were few choices of food and no nutrient-stripping processing.

They ate to survive. We eat because, well, jelly doughnuts.

Or whatever it is that tempts you. My current list of top temptations, which changes like stock prices: meatballs, pancakes, bacon cheeseburgers, tacos (various), Dairy Queen (all), peanut butter cups, whipped cream, icy coffee drinks, pretzel rolls, guacamole, and the finger food combo of onion and shredded cheese stuffed inside a black olive (eaten while preparing tacos). Oh, and a bagel with honey nut cream cheese. Are all these foods outright bad? Some would say yes unequivocally. Some would say, "Not if you don't have a lot of them." But if you fall among the latter set, you'd say that the problem isn't the food; it's that you can get it anytime, with zero restrictions. Eat however much you want. And for the love of big breakfasts, if a man wants some corned beef hash, a man is going to get some corned beef hash. Yet most of us aren't living a life in which we can eat whatever we want in whatever quantities we feel like and let either our metabolisms or our activities burn it all away.

A few years ago, I pitched a story to *Runner's World* magazine called "The Ultimate Guide to Pancakes." Seemed like a natural. Runners run. Runners eat. When runners run, they eat pancakes. The editors agreed, and I spent a few months in the syrup-drenched world of pancake making, pancake creating, and pancake pounding. As perhaps the largest of all the regular *Runner's World* writers—hence the title of *The Big Guy Blog*, which I write—I thought this assignment was a natural, but it also worried me. At the time, I had been trying to cut down on some carbs—I don't outright forbid them—and I simply didn't log the miles or have the speed to eat a lot of extras while trying to lose weight.

I traveled to Savannah, met up with a fun group, trotted out four miles, then had a morning meal at a place where the pancakes appeared to be the approximate size of a helipad. I left with a good sense of equilibrium—calories out, calories in. But then, about five miles into my drive home, I couldn't believe what I spotted: The Original Pancake House. And by "couldn't believe it," I mean "I may or may not have MapQuest directions there."

I lived near none of the more than one hundred Original Pancake House franchises around the country, but I had certainly heard of the OPH, and in the name of thorough research, I felt obligated to pull over and see what it was all about. Though my earlier cakes were still undigested, I looked at the OPH menu the way I would look at a wall of sneakers. I wanted all of them. So many colors. So many functions. How do I choose? Banana, peach, buckwheat, wheat germ, cinnamon-raisin, chocolate chip, blueberry, more, more, more . . .

"You ready to order?" the waitress asked.

My stomach was not ready to double-down on breakfast, but my curiosity was, so I asked, "Can I do a sampler or something?"

She glanced to the back of the restaurant in a way that looked as if I had just asked for the crack-flavored cakes and the cops were sitting two booths away.

"I think I can do that for you," she said in a hush, explaining that on a six-pancake plate, I can order three flavors, two each. "You just can't get anything that runs."

By this, she meant that I couldn't have any syrupy topping that would compromise the integrity of an adjacent pancake. But the only thing I could think of that wouldn't be able to run was me, after vacuuming up back-to-back breakfasts.

Since I didn't know which toppings would be off-limits, I made my selections and let my waitress guide me through.

"Can I have the bacon pancake?"

"Yes."

"Peanut butter?"

"Yep."

"Hmm, how about cinnamon-raisin?"

"I can do that."

She soon arrived with my plate. I tried a sample of each but, in what might be one of the only times in my life, did not finish my food. Granted, it was my second meal in an hour. If I had logged ten miles that morning, maybe I could have swung the two-fer. As I looked at that menu—all the choices, all the flavors, all the sweet goodness on the page—I couldn't help but think that this was exactly why fast food, processed food, junk food, and voluminous food were kicking and expanding our societal butts: The forbidden fruit is no longer forbidden, and it's no longer fruit.

Resistance Exercise: How to Deal with Temptation

The forces of temptation are like a strong ocean current: They wallop you like a wave, sweep you up, and carry you right out to the island of ninety-nine-cent burgers. Way too strong for you to swim your way out. Unlike other scenarios in which we think about temptation, food temptation doesn't have the perceived stigma of hurting someone else, as it does in, say, the case of adultery. So there's no moral influence on whether we give in to food temptations. So what if I have a fourth helping of scalloped potatoes, and then spend ten minutes scraping the bowl to get the last bit of crusted cheese off the pot? I'm not hurting anyone else, and I like crusted cheese. What's it to you? It's easier, and more satisfying in the moment, to succumb than to resist.

That served as the central question of early research involving the ideas of temptation, self-control, and delayed gratification. In the 1960s and '70s, psychologist Walter Mischel conducted the well-documented marshmallow experiment. In it, children were told they could have one marshmallow right now or two if they waited until the researcher came back into the room a short time later. Mischel tracked the children over time, and the short of it was that those who resisted temptation and didn't need the immediate gratification essentially had better life results (be it through work success, health, grades, and things of that nature). Being able to distract themselves so they wouldn't give in to the temptation, it appeared, served as some kind of marker for all kinds of coping skills. Note that this experiment has a flaw for the dieting set: The kid who waited still got the marshmallows, so there was a benefit to waiting. (The trouble with most diets is that the dieter resists, but doesn't get the marshmallows.)

Temptation (or impulse) is really considered one of our visceral, automatic responses as humans. It's in our nature to seek immediate gratification to those impulses. And most of us know the duh answer: Avoid the temptation. A Cambridge University study that largely examined the neurological mechanisms of self-control also showed what we already know. It's easier to avoid temptation if we're not exposed to it in the first place, than to resist a temptation that's right in front of us. (This study used heterosexual men tempted by various degrees of erotic photos.)

While it might be easy to say we can limit exposure to certain foods by not keeping them in our homes, we simply can't avoid the feeling of being tempted by our favorites when exposed to them—be it in the store, at the mall, in advertisements, any-where. So avoidance can't be the only answer, at least not in our current environment. This distinction is very important, says Eli Tsukayama, a postdoctoral fellow at the University of Pennsylvania who studies self-control. "As you can imagine, if we didn't have this impulse, we wouldn't have the problem in the first place," he said. "The impulses are automatic, but they depend on some kind of context, like somebody pisses you off, or how hungry you are, how long it's been since you've eaten, what you like as a person. Are you the kind of person who likes candy? I'm not a big fan of sweets, so for ice cream and cakes, I have relatively no temptation. But something like steak—I'm really tempted."

Instead of asking Tsukayama how he could not be a fan of ice cream, I asked him what would drive those differences—why some of us seem to have more self-control than others. It's sus-pected, as with just about every other factor to do with obesity, that the reason involves some mix of genetics, culture, environ-ment, and what our parents exposed us to as we were forming our tastes and preferences. The self-control research, whether it in-volves food or money, usually points to people choosing smaller rewards sooner than the possibility of a larger reward down the line. "In almost all self-control research, the question is, 'Would I prefer immediate pleasure of eating this now or the delayed out-come of being healthy or being strong or being thin?' That's not as tangible and not as exciting as in the moment," Tsukayama said.

So if the automatic response is to give into temptation, how are we supposed to deal with chicken parm sandwiches? What is the fight? What chance do we even stand?

Some would argue that the issue isn't necessarily about the strength of wills—i.e., if you can just stare down the goo-filled baked good right into its smarmy little cream hole, then you will outmuscle it and beat it. Some would argue that it comes down to creating environments that minimize temptations, such as by not keeping junk food in the house. Some would argue that changing your habits can work, too, so that your automatic response becomes more powerful than the impulse to give in every time you see a caramel-flavored treat. So instead of having dessert after dinner, you have a cup of coffee with a touch of sweetener in it, which can satisfy sweet cravings, occupy your tongue, and distract your mind at a fraction of the calories. Even in as quickly as a few weeks, behavior specialists say, you can create a new habit to override the unhealthy impulses. Another lesson comes in those early marshmallow studies: Distraction techniques can work by getting you out of the danger zone. The kids who had success (that is, those who waited until the researcher returned to the room after about fifteen minutes), compared to those who gave in either right away or after a few minutes, were able to distract themselves by thinking that the items in front of them were not marshmallows but rather clouds or cotton balls. Work done by Roy Baumeister, PhD, an eminent scholar at Florida State University, shows that self-control works a lot like a muscle: The more you work it, the stronger it gets. And vice versa: The less you use self-control, the more likely you are to give in to temptation.

In one of his studies published in the *European Journal of Personality*, Tsukayama summarized the plight of Tiger Woods and noted the paradox of his being lauded for his mental discipline when it came to golf, but (by his own admission) not having any self-control when it came to extramarital sex. In the study, Tsukayama and his team conducted experiments to test the conditions under which individuals were more likely to give in to temptation. One finding: Individuals were more likely to resist temptations that had harmful effects. That conclusion summarizes the weight struggle for many people. We know that eating unhealthily can cause bad things to happen, but the harms are not immediate in the way that not wearing a seat belt might be, so we rationalize that our behaviors are not all that risky. (Tsukayama speculated that Woods's actions may have been driven by the fact that he didn't think he could be caught, so he didn't see the harmful effects of his actions.) This is called "temporal discounting," the tendency to devalue a harmful thing according to its distance from us in time. The further away in time it is, the less importance we give it. We have steeper discount rates for rewards that we desire and enjoy more. If you take away the morality issues at play—I know this is a big *if*—you can look at Woods's menu of other women as not unlike the menus we're tempted with every day. Lots of options, lots of temptations; choose whatever you like whenever you like.

We often think of willpower as being about suffering. I can stick to the plan, no matter how much it hurts. I can resist the doughnut even if you put it in front of me. It's about strength. Except it's not. Stanford psychologist Kelly McGonigal, PhD, author of *The Willpower Instinct*, who teaches a course in the area, has said that we can develop willpower skills. It's more about strategy than grit or impulses. While we can't control what we think and feel, we can control what we do—which is where strategy comes into play. In her work, she has explained that we can better equip our brains to resist temptations by doing things like setting goals, getting sleep and food (to fuel our brains with enough energy to make decisions), and even setting up a rewards system that will help us avoid the evil temptation and replace it with something that can still satisfy our cravings—which may just serve as the most important temptation-resisting tactic of all.

Solution: Flowchart the Cheese Sauce

There's a category of people I've always admired: people who are cool as Popsicles in an emergency. Lifeguards, paramedics, ER personnel, military folks—you name it. Trouble strikes, they react, do their jobs, save a life. I imagine many would tell you the reason they don't panic is partly because of their personalities, but it's also because of their training: They have a plan, they know the process, they've practiced. It's an emergency to everyone involved—except for those who are calming it down and fixing the problem. I don't want to flippantly compare life-and-death accidents and rescue missions to a tabletop of tortilla chips, but the lesson still holds. The one thing we can do to better equip ourselves for dietary emergencies is to have a plan in place, then employ that plan when we need it.

Peter Gollwitzer, PhD, a professor of psychology at New York University who studies goals and how emotions, cognition, and behaviors influence them, said that when talking about the ability to resist temptation, context is extremely important. In the United

States especially, we're up against a formidable opponent in that it's easy (and encouraged) to eat a lot and eat poorly. In this kind of environment, you need a lot of self-regulatory skills. "Some people are born with them. And some have more than others, like intelligence," Gollwitzer said. Those skills, like any other, can be developed. The first step: articulating goals and creating a plan to get there. How are you going to reach your goal? The next step is just as crucial. When things get tough, how do you stay on track, how do you continue to get to your goal, how do you make good choices when things don't go well? How do you resist temptation?

One thing Gollwitzer told me stood out: Losing weight is not that difficult. "It's not like inventing a new type of car or something like that."

Losing weight is not that difficult? For many of us, it feels like the hardest thing we've ever had to do. What I suspect he meant is that there's plenty of information available about how to lose weight, and most of us know there's a huge difference nutritionally between, say, zucchini and fried zucchini sticks. We're not lacking in information. We're not lacking the cognitive skills to understand what we tend to do right with our diets and what we don't. We just don't *do*. To create the bridge from *know* to *do*, all it takes is two more words.

If and *then*.

This is the emergency response plan: If *x* happens, you do *y*.

So when you create the plan about losing weight, along with the steps on how you're going to do it, the next step is creating "if and then" scenarios to help you with your most common temptation. If your coworkers ask you to happy hour every Thursday, then what? If the server brings out bread that you know you shouldn't pick at, then what? If your partner pours a bowl of Lucky Charms every night, then what? Create a mental (or actual) list of the scenarios most likely to derail you. What will happen is that your *then* will start to become habit. Offered a drink, you say, "No, thanks. I'll have one tomorrow." Partner eating blocks of cheese? That's your cue to get the veggies and hummus. These simple responses and action plans are typically enough to stave off the temptation, the in-the-moment impulse, and help you stick to your plan for achieving your main goals. Your contingency plan means you override the impulse you may have to say, "Sure, why not? What's one gin and tonic going to hurt?" (when you know it may lead to four).

If-then is what keeps showing up in studies as an effective strategy, because it's a simple and instant way to break habits, Gollwitzer said. When you're faced with frustration or temptation that goes against the spirit of your goal, the if-then statement shoots up to the top of your mind. Your automatic response grows into whatever your articulated *then* statement is, rather than you reflexively diving into a meringue pie.

I'm not against meringue pie or any other treat, but dealing with temptation is about dealing with *chronic* temptation. Many of us operate best in a system that allows us to enjoy the foods we love and crave, even if they aren't officially part of any particular diet plan. (More on this in chapter 7.) I believe that creating some kind of "out"—be it small portions of whatever sin food you love, or a cheat meal once a week—helps stave off chronic temptations. The tactic Gollwitzer suggests serves as the perfect strategy for dealing with the big picture of self-control; it's not about making a commitment to giving up everything forever, but it gives you tangible actions. Rather than articulating the goal ("I'm going to eat healthy"), you have a specific plan ("If my husband orders dessert, then I will have two bites").

One of the best ways I've heard of for dealing with the so-called tempting foods came from Liam McIntyre, the actor who plays the lead role in the Starz series *Spartacus*. I interviewed him for a story for *Men's Health*, about his training. For his role, he often appeared nearly naked and needed to look strong and lean, a serious motivating factor undoubtedly. When I asked him about his nutrition, he said he ate as well as possible (lean meats, vegetables, healthy fats), except during one two-hour window a week. During that window, he could eat whatever he wanted and as much as he wanted; he chose pizza and baked goods most of the time. It turned out that he often felt sick after doing so, because he had been eating so well the rest of the week. Indulging like this served as that once-a-week carrot that looked nothing like a carrot. McIntyre obviously had a special incentive for looking good: He was on camera, and this was his job. For the rest of us who don't need to bare our bodies in front of millions, that kind of cheat strategy is a perfect example of Gollwitzer's if-then tactic. If somebody wants to go out with you for pizza, choose that as your cheat meal. If you get asked to do it Wednesday, Thursday, *and* Friday, say you're doing it Saturday. That strategy allows you to stick to the plan and steer yourself clear of chronic temptations—without having to give up all of them. When Gollwitzer and his colleague did a meta-analysis of ninety-four studies on the use of if-then strategies (involving more than eight thousand people), called "intention implementation," they found the strategy had a moderate to large effect on people's attainment of goals.

After I talked to Gollwitzer, I tried a few if-then statements to help me navigate through danger zones. If my family wants to go out for Mexican, then I order a grilled chicken salad as my main dish. (That way, I can order one taco and have a few heavily salsa'd chips but don't blow my whole meal on high-goo Mexican food.) If I meet my friends for a beer, then I order a beer and water (to slow down my drinking and essentially cut my beers to two, rather than risk having three or four). If I *have* to have Dairy Queen, then I tell myself I have to wait until a day when I've exercised for more than an hour. (This delays the impulsive reaction and also means I'm less likely to want the ice cream when the time comes.)

What this tactic does is essentially take the person from a "hot" state to a "cold" state. A Northwestern University study by Loran F. Nordgren and Eileen Y. Chou found that when people were in a "cold," or nonvisceral, state, they were better able to use self-control against temptation than when they were in a "hot," visceral, state. This hot state comes about when our bodies feel the urge to satisfy some basic need, like hunger or thirst, so our brains make decisions that support short-term goals. The cold state happens when our needs are essentially satisfied and we can use our brains to override those impulses to make decisions that include not just short-term satisfaction but also long-term goals. In one experiment, these researchers looked at heterosexual men's attention and sexual arousal in response to attractive women; in another, they used smoking as the temptation. So the takeaway? As dieters dealing with temptations, we have to find ways of not being constantly in a hot state, where a short-term hunger or craving makes us more likely to give in to whatever food is available to us, rather than to think through and make a choice about what might be best for us. It's the classic case of taking a cold shower, except, instead of pouring cold water on your body parts, you're dumping it on your worst food triggers. In a study published in the *Journal of Consumer Research*, researchers found that subtle word choice can be effective in helping us make better food choices—that is, "I don't" is more effective than "I can't." So it was an issue of empowerment—the sense that "I don't eat ice cream" gives more control to the person than "I can't eat ice cream." In one of the experiments, subjects were told to practice one of the two phrases in relation to tempting, unhealthy foods. They filled out a questionnaire, and when they turned it in, they were given a choice between taking a chocolate candy bar or a granola bar. (Note: Granola bars aren't necessarily healthy, though people have the perception of their being healthier than candy.) The researchers found that those assigned to the "I don't" group chose the granola bar 64 percent of the time, while those in the "I can't" group chose it only 39 percent of the time.

Without even knowing it, I used this tactic in the way I approached kicking a two-decade-old addiction to diet soda. It involves a subtle word change, but one that seems to take the edge off temptation. No diet plan is telling you what to do. You're simply making a choice about what you are and aren't eating.

When Can You Give In?

Chris Garcia didn't gain the "freshman fifteen." He gained seventy-five. The summer after his junior year, he had a blood pressure of 206/120 and needed to be hospitalized for a week. "I was at risk of having a stroke at that point—a week before my twenty-first birthday. That was eye-opening," he said. After that, he went on the Atkins diet and lost 50 pounds, but then he met a girl, so he thought, "Okay, my work here is done," and gained 40 of it back and ended up graduating college at 350 pounds.

Chris came from a family with eating problems; his father's side of the family was very large, and his mom had eating issues, too. Chris always gravitated toward finger foods, food he could just pick at and pick at and pick at, whether it was a bag of chips or all-you-can-eat chicken wings. Food was something he went to when he was bored; it was also problematic because of all the social interactions that happen around food. (His friends are thin and eat anything they want.)

Two years ago, he decided to give weight loss another shot. He joined Weight Watchers, began to run, and started practicing a Brazilian martial art called capoeira. His weight gradually decreased, and he worked his way down to 265 pounds. He dropped from a size 46 in jeans to a size 38. "I don't remember ever having a pair of pants with a three in it," he said.

The biggest thing for Chris was the support of his friends (and of strangers) in his capoeira class. "Whether it's silly or not, it seemed like they were invested in me doing well," he said. "If I had at all felt like they were judging me or I didn't feel accepted, I would've quit in the first week."

Without knowing he was doing so, he also used the exact techniques that help us resist chronic temptations: One, he distracted himself. He signed up for a running race without ever having run three miles in his life. He used that experience to keep him looking for more. He'd spend hours a day on the Internet, talking with friends about new goals, new races, and new experiences. "I just kept signing up [for races], and if I'm going to spend money on these, I'm going to do it," he said. "It became an addiction: looking up races, looking up gear, looking up what diets people are on for running. I thought, 'If I'm going to be addicted to anything, it might as well be exercise.'" Two, he came up with strategies to help him cope with temptations that came along when socializing with his friends. For example, he ate before he went out (thus putting himself in that cold state, and also doing a form of if-then: "If my friends go out, then I will eat before we go"). He adjusted his thinking to order healthier items by telling himself that he needed to fuel himself better for the activities he enjoyed doing, rather than simply satisfy cravings.

Chris wants to get down to 230 pounds and gain some muscle. Also, he has signed up for other kinds of races, including a half marathon, and learned how to manage temptations so he doesn't have to give up his favorite foods forever. "I do know what I'm going to eat after the half marathon," Chris said. "Chicken wings." Chris found the balance he needed: eating healthy most of the time, and then picking windows during which he could have the foods he used to live on.

For my most recent weight-loss success, I used that tactic often: eating healthy as much as possible, but enjoying treats from time to time. (Some argue with this line of thinking.) And as of now, I have no off-limits foods. Except one: diet soda.

When I met my wife, she drank Diet Coke. I didn't drink much soda, but when I did, it was the regular kind. As my weight started to increase, I made the decision to switch from regular to diet. Easy, right? Nothing wrong with something that's zero calories. Not sure I can think of a better deal.

It took a little while to get used to the taste of diet drinks, and I can't tell you when the switch morphed into an all-out addiction. Soon I was drinking Diet Coke with every meal and using it as a snack to curb cravings—and likely subconsciously to justify other, unhealthier choices. I drank it, or a variation of it—diet cream soda!—all the time. And I never once saw *that* as contributing to my weight problem. Zero calories couldn't be the cause. Then more and more research came out about how diet drinks could actually be part of the problem. One research review from Purdue University found that artificially sweetened drinks may put people at risk of weight gain, cardiovascular disease, and type 2 diabetes. The thinking goes that these artificial beverages don't induce the chemical and hormonal effects that do things like curb hunger or keep you satisfied. Still, the review concluded that other factors were also in play, since not everyone with a weight problem drinks artificially sweetened beverages. But the evidence mounted. In recent research by the University of Texas, the results were staggering: Those who consumed more than two diet drinks a day had waist size increases six times greater than those who didn't. To be fair, diet drinks are better for people who drink a lot of high-sugar drinks, and some would argue that the research is still very preliminary on how much, if any, influence diet drinks have on weight gain (or not helping with weight loss).

I don't know why I decided to pick on my Diet Coke addiction, or why I decided to declare that my relationship with it was over, since I had never done that with any other food. But on July 6, 2011—I remember it as if it were a first-day sobriety date—I decided to give it up, and frankly, I've been tempted to drink it only a few times since then. After the first few days, I never really missed it. Part of the reason for this, even though I didn't know it at the time, was that I transferred my state from hot to cold: I had never had to rely on Diet Coke to satisfy my thirst, and simply made the decision that water would do just as well. I also decided to look at why I had needed Diet Coke so much in the first place, and I realized that while I did like the taste, my addiction was more about the habit—about having something slightly sweet, about always having something on my desk to sip while writing. So I did what I think was the key to making a meaningful change, and I did some of the things that have been shown to work. I replaced my Diet Coke habit with the much healthier option of water and/or coffee. So what if I (say the next word slowly) *occasionally* use Almond Joy–flavored creamer?

I used this important strategy when it came to behavior change: I didn't *not* do something, cutting something out without replacing it. Instead, I dropped one drink for another. That way, I never felt I was in a hot state, and I always felt that I could give my brain an action to perform.

As of this writing, I've been diet drink–free for three years, except for a rogue sip I accidently took of my wife's drink and swallowed before I realized what it was. I don't drink it anymore— not that I *can't*; I *don't*.

I don't know why this diet-drink research struck me more than any other, and I don't know exactly why it's the only temptation I've decided to banish outright. It was probably because I drank so much of it that it was the only food I couldn't have just a little of; everything else, I have no problem with handling in moderation. Just as I had deemed diet drinks to be the answer to thwarting my weight gain some twenty years ago, I decided that they were quite possibly part of the problem. I can't remember ever having been successful at cold turkey. For the most part, I think abrupt (and a declaration of permanent) change sets us up for failure. Or at least it does me. Maybe I had some success because it was only one small change and not a whole slew of them at one time. Maybe it was because I needed to prove to myself that there was one thing I could hunker down and do, and this would be a manageable way of doing so. This time, cold turkey worked. Cold turkey, by the way, is best served on a roll with stuffing and cranberry. Made by a sub shop called Capriotti's where I grew up in Delaware, this righteous concoction is called The Bobbie. I would humbly suggest to Capriotti's to add a thin layer of mashed potatoes to The Bobbie. For this, I would happily, yet only occasionally, give in to temptation. But just once in a very long while.

Truth: Focusing on Process Will Get You Unstuck

Living about two hours from the Atlantic Ocean, we have to leave the house early if my twin boys want any chance of surfing some smallish summer morning waves. On the days we go, we load the boys' boards into my wife's Ford F-250 diesel pickup truck. (Liz is an equestrian, so she needs the truck for hauling hay and towing a trailer.)

One morning before 8:00 a.m., when only a few walkers dotted the beach, I put the truck into four-wheel drive and rolled onto the sand. As I turned to park, we stopped—and sank.

I tried going forward. I tried going in reverse. I told the boys to start digging around the tires to see if we could create some space so I could creep out. Nothing worked. And then the truck sank so deeply that the bed, which usually comes up to my waist, fell to ankle height.

Since we were losing wave time, I told the boys (then about ten or eleven) to get their boards and go. Not a surfer but always having wanted to be one, I walked to the shoreline to watch over them, leaving the truck a couple of hundred feet away as a public symbol of my idiocy. Soon, more people came to the beach. One man, who had seen my struggles from afar, walked over and said, "Yeah, I was surprised you took that big, heavy diesel out here."

I didn't know what I was going to do, but I resigned myself to the fact that the only answer would involve a towing vehicle, embarrassment, and a "Really?" from Liz when I returned home. When my boys took a break from the water, I tried one more time. Forward, reverse, dig. Forward, reverse, dig. Nothing. I tried to muscle this six-thousand-pound machine out of the earth, and the only direction it went was down.

As the lifeguards came on duty a couple of hours later, one saw the truck and walked over. He asked me if I had switched the hubs.

"Uh?" I grunted.

He bent down, turned a couple latches on the front two tires, and told me to put the truck in Drive and step on the gas.

I did as instructed, and I rolled out of the sand as if I were parked on blacktop. I then zipped up to the safety of the parking lot to avoid a second sand swallowing. My first thought: That lifeguard just saved me some money and some face.

I also had a second thought, sometime later: For so many of us, this is exactly what the whole weight-loss problem is about.

The Soul of Stuck: Might Doesn't Matter

The time I spent trapped in the sand felt similar to the way my whole adult life has felt, only measured in decades, not hours. We take actions that maybe we don't think are all that risky, and then one day we find ourselves stuck, spinning our wheels, frustrated, desperate for a solution. Maybe it's seeing a photograph, maybe it's getting a bad blood-pressure reading, maybe it's that we can't fit into our clothes anymore. Now we regret the decisions we've made—it would have been easier to avoid the pizza in the first place—yet we're stuck in the sand. We move forward, we dig in as hard as we can, we muscle our way to a new body with a complete and drastic diet and fitness overhaul—new book, new gym membership, new plan, new outlook. We're going to beat the pepperoni out of the obesity epidemic with a fifty-pound bag of baby carrots. It must work, it has to work, just a little harder, a little harder, and this scale is finally going to move in the right direction. It works for a bit, but then we plateau, and the things that have worked now stop working. So the hole just grows bigger and bigger and bigger. At the same time, people around you are surfing the waves of life—and doing what *you* want to be doing. Others are staring and judging your actions: *Yeah, I was surprised that you stuck that big, heavy diesel piece of lasagna in your mouth.*

My whole life, I'd dig in, then fall back. I'd feel good for a while and then I'd think, "Really, Dairy Queen has a S'Mores Blizzard?" The hole, and my pants, kept growing bigger.

It took me a while to figure out that the message from my truck-in-the-sand experience wasn't just to read the stinking driver's manual or to Google "dumbass stuck big truck on beach." The real lesson came from how we got the truck out of the sand, in the form of the lifeguard who solved my problem in about four seconds: The answer was in front of us the whole time, but it took someone else to unlock it. Is this how we get unstuck? Look somewhere you haven't looked? Trust others to help you? The best solution isn't about how mighty you are.

I have a friend, Doug Newburg, who has taught me some life-changing lessons about the notions of "feel" (which I'll explain in a few chapters). He's essentially a performance coach, a PhD psychologist who has studied the experiences of elite performers and everyday people and how they not only achieve success, but also create the lives that they want. Over many a lunch, I tried explaining my weight issues to him—what I did, why I did it. I would go on and on, talking about all the cool exercises I'd been doing; how I played hoops, lifted weights, and ran. "I do all this," I would say, "but I'm also so frustrated because the needle never seems to move. And when it does, it's always in the up direction." I *knew* I was doing the right things. I didn't do everything perfectly, but I knew enough about food and exercise that I should at least have seen some progress. One day, Doug just half-chuckled, and then explained that he sees the same situation all the time—not just in weight, but in careers, in athletics, in homes, in all arenas of life. It's the exact problem with anyone who ever feels stuck.

"If it's not working," he said, "then why do you keep doing the same thing?"

His message, which sounded simple, was about power: We think we can will our way to where we want to go if we have determination. We tell ourselves that if we just press harder on the gas, things will work out. If we try harder, if we push harder, if we just take care of business, then we will succeed. In fact, that's what may be making us sink deeper and deeper. To get where you want—to lose weight, to break through a plateau, to stop the frustration that comes along with spinning your wheels—it's not necessarily about a major overhaul. It's about finding the hub in your life that you can unlock to get you unstuck.

The Answer: Process, Not Results

Since the 1930s, researchers have been studying the link between frustration and aggression with essentially this conclusion: If someone blocks you from achieving a goal, there's a tendency to respond with aggression toward that person. Not surprising, right? We see it all the time—whether it's road rage or a hockey fight or lashing out at a spouse. The source of the frustration doesn't have to come in the form of a dingbat driver or a husband who never wipes down the wet glasses from the dishwasher before putting them in the cabinet. The source can also come from in-animate objects—a tree falling in the roadway and blocking traf-fic. Brad Bushman, PhD, a professor of communication and psychology at Ohio State University who studies human aggres-sion, defined the relationship as one that certainly applies to weight loss: "Anything that blocks your goal increases your ten-dency to lash out, often against innocent victims." What happens when *you're* your own roadblock? It's even harder to find your way around it, because you direct your aggression to the fifth shelf in the pantry.

This is especially true, Bushman said, when you experience chronic levels of frustration because of the "no end in sight" men-tality, in which you don't anticipate an imminent solution (a way around the tree, a shortcut to losing the weight). Bushman said that we all essentially have two responses when faced with frus-tration. Aggression is the most maladaptive response, he said, adding that it's also the most natural one. Evolutionarily, there must have been a reason that acting aggressively helped us. Frus-trated that you're surrounded by three lions and you need to get dinner back to the family? Reasoning won't help, so aggression may be your only way to get around the problem. It's played out in today's society, too. The first thing to do when faced with frustration is to lash out: hit, punch, yell, kick. "It's the worst thing you can do," Bushman said, "but it's what comes naturally." So what we see, psychologically, is that when stress levels are very high (or also very low, for that matter), we revert to the way we'd act naturally. We don't think; we act. "Under stress, you rely on what you already know how to do," Bushman said. In that case, we've then done nothing actually to solve the problem at hand.

The adaptive approach, of course, is the exact opposite of aggression: Use your cognitive resources to figure out what's going on, Bushman said.

This is why the clichéd "take a walk" and "take deep breaths" solutions to stress and frustration work. They give your stress response (your instinctual response) time to calm down and let your brain come up with a solution to your obstacle. True, taking deep breaths while staring down a can of SpaghettiOs may help get you out of that immediate jam of canned calories. But those of us who struggle with feeling stuck in an unhealthy weight have to find a way to change the bigger picture when it comes to our maladaptive responses—be they aggression or depression or anxiety, or using whole pies to make us feel better for not feeling better. In that case, we have to use the "deep breath" symbolism to give our brains a chance to help our bodies—that is, it's not a momentary breath in the face of a candy bar, but rather the act of stepping away from the issues to figure out answers. Our brains (using such cognitive resources) can figure out the solution if we give them a chance to do so.

As chronic weight gainers and losers, we can draw some

lessons from the world of sports performance. I once watched a video by sports psychology expert Patrick Cohn, PhD, about how athletes become frustrated with their performance in youth sports. He broke it down this way: For an athlete who's experiencing frustration, there are two important concepts, the trigger and the emotions. The trigger is some kind of action on the field: a poor play, a missed shot, a mental mistake, or a cheating opponent. And the emotion is the consequence of that trigger: anger, frustration, or helplessness. One leads directly to the other, except—and this is a big except—there's a whole chasm between the trigger and emotion. Cohn argues that this chasm is filled with beliefs. For the athlete, what is the belief? That others will think you're bad if you make a mistake, that you have to be perfect?

Sounds exactly the way dieters think. "What will the world think of me when I need to buy two airplane seats?" "What if I order the burger and fries and eat the whole thing?" "Will my spouse think I'm a slob if I keep gaining weight?" "What is the consequence of slamming down a football-size burrito?"

To change the emotions, it takes shifting beliefs. For youth sports, it may be teaching kids that mistakes are okay—everyone makes them; that's the nature of sports, since there's no such thing as perfection, except maybe in bowling and gymnastics. But how do we do it as adults? How do we take something as embedded in our minds as our beliefs about body and weight and flip them upside down? How do we tell ourselves that mistakes are okay when we know full well that mac-and-cheese omelets are *not* a health food? How do we tell ourselves that the goal isn't perfection, but rather the blander "being good most of the time"? The argument would go that you're not going to be able to limit your triggers. (There will always be 4,000-calorie doughnut concoctions, just as there will always be pressure to make free throws at the end of the game.) But you can change your response to those triggers, if you can change what you believe to be true about weight loss and dieting. While not a weight-loss expert, Cohn makes a good point that can be applied to this subject: The way to improve composure, he told me, is that you have to differentiate between expectations and goals. People get frustrated when they don't meet their expectation that they have to eat perfectly at every meal. While it's good to have goals, he said, it's more important to manage your expectations of how you *should* perform. By focusing on the process instead of the final number, you're more likely to get to the outcome you want. "If you do the process well," he said, "that will eventually lead to the desired outcomes. Focus on the execution—in athletics, it's shot-to-shot or pitch-to-pitch execution—knowing that if you focus on doing the action well, the result will take care of itself. But if you're so obsessed with reaching a weight-loss goal, does that help you do the process? That's backward. It doesn't help you get to the outcome."

In practice, this means you keep the desired weight or that pair of skinny jeans as the goal, but you stop *focusing on them*. Instead, shift your attention to whatever process you're going to use to get there. And when things don't go right, you also have to manage your mistakes, not beat yourself up about them. That, of course, takes some practice and the ability to work through the frustrations of scale numbers not moving or body shapes not changing.

Here's an interesting side note about the development of those goals: In the mainstream media, we've been pounded with the message that we need to set reasonable goals; if you have a better shot at attaining a goal, the argument goes, you're more likely to succeed. However, a recent paper examining obesity myths, published in *The New England Journal of Medicine*, challenged this notion. The authors pointed to several studies, including one in the journal *Obesity*, showing that those who articulated a dream weight were positively correlated to weight loss over the long term—and that there was no significant correlation between realistic weight goals and actual weight loss. Matthew Herper, who wrote about the *NEJM* paper for *Forbes*, made a good point: "I'm a great believer in clinical trials, but it's always important to remember that just because a clinical trial does not show an effect doesn't mean that effect doesn't exist." That means that those of us who are challenged with these struggles have to gather evidence in all forms (studies, stories, experimentation)—not figure out the recipe that will unequivocally work, but to find the one that will give us the best chance for succeeding, for breaking through plateaus, for working through the inevitable frustration we encounter.

Art Markman, PhD, a professor of psychology and marketing at the University of Texas at Austin and author of the book *Smart Change*, studies such things as decision making, goals, and motivation. He said that part of the reason weight loss is so difficult and frustrating is because our brains are not wired to handle the absence of action.

"When you're trying to lose weight, you're trying to eat less, avoid certain tempting foods," he told me. "If you succeed, if you achieve that negative goal, what you've done is *not* doing something. The problem with not doing something is that your brain basically doesn't learn not to do something. When every time you've successfully resisted a pint of Ben & Jerry's, you've achieved something significant, but your brain really hasn't changed. What you have to do in order to be really successful is turn all these negative goals into positive ones—actions that you're going to take in particular circumstances, actions and things you can learn to do."

That made a lot of sense: Most of our struggles come from the fact that we're deleting content from our brains, rather than trying to upload new files for our brains to work on. It also makes sense when combined with Cohn's take on the process: that is, laser-beaming our attention on the process, whether it's writing down what you eat, logging the miles you walk, or aiming to eat nine fruits or vegetables a day. But if your tactic is just to deny yourself x, y, and z, then your brain will soon enter a sort of emergency state. An empty mind, after all, will go back to what it knows, a.k.a. meatball subs. In a way, to shift out of bad eating habits, it's not as much about denying ourselves or resisting or having the mental grit to fight the aroma of snickerdoodles. It's much more about keeping our brains fat and happy. Another interesting note: One experiment about frustration involved denying rats sweetened water. Research shows that the rats who express less anxiety over levels of frustration are those in groups, rather than ones in isolation, a theme that comes up time and time again.

Addition Equals Subtraction

In the year or so after Mary Weil's parents' divorce when she was in middle school, she gained somewhere in the neighborhood of a hundred pounds. When the divorce happened, her life changed. Instead of coming home after school and playing, she'd have to go to her grandmother's house, where she'd just sit around. Her father was now in charge of some meals, and he would always order pizza or cook up chicken nuggets. When her eating and activity habits changed, her body ballooned. She entered college at 307 pounds and graduate school at 325. At that point, she lost 25, but then got caught up in her studies and gained it all back, graduating at 345 pounds.

"It was tough because I had always seen weight loss as an unattainable thing, this huge project that would take so long," she told me. Mary, who documents her journey on the blog *A Small Loss*, spent years frustrated. She tried SlimFast shakes and popular weight-loss pills and restrictive diets, but she'd always find a way around whatever the given program wanted her to do. "If you say, 'You can't do this,' I'm the kind of personality that will just obsess about it. Especially after my parents' divorce, I had a lot of binge-eating tendencies, and I used food as comfort," she said. "I still struggle with my food. If I'm told I can't have it, I can crave it intensely until I binge on it."

Mary hit her bottom moments before her master's exams (those periods of high stress). She bought fifty dollars' worth of junk food—while not classically defined as aggressive, this could be interpreted as the maladaptive response to frustration—gorged on it, and got sick.

"I bought these cookies that looked like watermelon and didn't realize what they tasted like," she said. "And they were disgusting, but I ate them anyway. I bought two boxes because they were adorable. And I ate so many of them."

Soon after that moment, and coinciding with graduation, it all sort of clicked. Her family had come to visit, and Mary was exhausted from all the sightseeing. When she went back home to visit, she took twenty-four hours' worth of train journeys, rather than an hour-and-a-half plane flight, because she didn't want to be stuck in the middle seat of an airplane. She realized something had to give.

Mary decided it was the perfect time to lose weight, and her parents bought her a Wii Fit. Initially, she exceeded the weight limit to use the video game scale and platform, so she had to lose fifteen pounds before she could even start with that program. To do that, she started walking around the block and getting off the bus a few stops early. "It was literally all I could do," she said. She started making dietary changes: cutting out sodas and eating foods that were as minimally processed as possible. She did as many little things as she could—eventually signing up for a charity walk with coworkers. Then she put a big goal on her calendar: Though she knew she couldn't run it, she wanted to do something in conjunction with the Chicago Marathon. So she decided that because her office had twenty-six floors, she would aim to walk up her entire building on marathon day. She started her training with a few floors, then more. Then, on the day of the marathon, she raced up the whole building. "All these girls in the office couldn't do the stairs, and I'm the big girl in the office, and I did it," she said.

Her race coincided with a fifty-pound loss—and nobody at work even noticed.

"It was unbelievable. Finally, later, someone said to me one day, 'Have you lost weight?' and I said, 'Yeah, I've lost seventy-five pounds. It took you that long to realize it?'"

Mary got down to 188 pounds, and while she's bounced back up after having a baby, she attributes her ability to work past her frustrations to several factors: making those small changes and focusing on the process, having a husband who understands (he's lost almost a hundred pounds himself), making routines rather than having restrictions (she treats herself to Lean Cuisine pizza once a week as a treat), and using her blog as a way both to give and to receive support.

"When I'm struggling—and it always seems to work this way—and I have a really rough night and don't want to work out or cook up chicken, I'd rather order a pizza instead. That's when you get an e-mail that says, 'What you said changed my life. I'm staring up the same mountain and have a hundred and fifty pounds to lose. If Mary can do it, I can do it, too.'"

I know a bit how Mary has felt when it comes to frustration, to feeling stuck in a body that you're not happy with. During my adult life, I've lost more than forty pounds a couple of times. One of my best performances came in 1993. I had ballooned to 231 pounds, seemingly from a new work schedule and the social life that came with it. *Why, yes, I will play on the company softball team. Oh, it involves postgame beverages and jalapeño poppers? How nice.* I knew I needed to lose weight, but I was still fairly active, so I tended to ignore the warning signs that my weight was creeping up.

Until one weekend in October.

Liz and I decided to sign up for a charity bike event, one in which we'd cycle seventy-five miles to the beach on a Saturday and then seventy-five miles back on Sunday. We were about a year into our relationship at the time and thought it'd be a fun weekend. (Weeks into our relationship, we also thought it would be fun to go for runs together—a mile to the convenience store, to pick up a pint of ice cream, and then a mile back. I soon learned that my burn-and-consume calorie equation was slightly off.) We had only fat-tire mountain bikes, so we knew our speeds would be naturally slower than those on zippy road bikes. Saturday started fine, but as the day progressed, so did the headwinds. We pedaled but didn't go very fast; stopping at every rest stop slowed our progress. By the time we rolled in, our legs were cooked, and I had serious saddle sores in cracks and crevices that I'm not sure I knew humans had.

We dreaded the ride home, but hoped the headwinds turned to tailwinds on Sunday. Morning came, and we left an hour before everybody else, to try to get a jump on the pack. My butt sores burned so much that I balled up a pair of Liz's underwear and stuffed them down my pants in an attempt to add padding to my cycle seat. This did not work well.

We grinded for hours. With ten miles left, I felt as if I were cycling into a wall—my legs hurt, the wind stiffened, few bikes were left on the course. Liz charged forward, but I struggled. Even though I wanted to give other explanations for why I sucked (headwinds, fat tires), I knew why: I was too damn big. When I got home, I weighed myself. I had gained five pounds over the weekend. I had gained five pounds. After. Cycling. One hundred and fifty miles.

How many rest stop cookies did I actually have?

In the following week, I concocted a plan, which involved eating better, running, and lifting weights—nothing surprising in the realm of solutions. But to this day, I think the central component as to why I was able to lose weight during that stretch was an indoor track that measured one-twenty-second of a mile and overlooked a basketball court at my gym. Crazy small. Most runners would rather pop blood blisters than have to hamster-wheel their runs on a track that size. For me, I could tick off the laps quickly, even if I moved slowly. Instead of counting by mile, I could count up to one hundred, down from one hundred, ten sets of ten, three slow and then three fast—whatever it was that would help me go a little bit longer or be a little bit stronger. I focused on process. I focused on small things that would add up quickly. A couple of laps turned into a couple of miles. I used an answer that was right in front of me but that I had never tried before. I filled my brain with something *to do*, rather than with something *to eat*. I didn't try to outmuscle my frustrations, just outsmart them. I know most people would lose their sanity before dedicating time to running consistently on a track that size—and I'm not implying that this in particular is the answer that will work for everyone (or anyone, for that matter). The point is that I found the solution of adding up little victories that would result in a big one. (The other thing that played a role: I upgraded my membership so I could use the steam room after my workouts.)

I hit my goal and lost forty pounds within about four months. By making me concentrate on every little lap rather than the number waiting for me at the end, that track helped me find my way out. It was one of the few times in my life when I felt stuck deep in the sand and was able to figure out how to break free.

Truth: If You're the Butt of a Joke, You Must Then Kick Butt

Though I had a well-earned rep of being slower and wider than most runners (especially by the standards of my lean and fit *Men's Health* magazine coworkers at the time), I had trained diligently for my first half marathon. A little over thirty years old and hovering in the 210-pound range (downright slim compared to the weight I would see a few years later), I ran five days a week with two buddies from the office. I followed a plan created by an elite marathoner. I didn't blaze my miles, but I logged them. The only thing that went wrong during the months-long program: During the two weeks before the race, I felt burned out and could barely muster one or two final trots. My tapering period (the time before a long race when you're supposed to reduce your effort so you're fresh for race day) felt more like a meltdown. Still, I believed, I had run faithfully and earned a solid, if not superspeedy, race.

The morning of the race, I felt good through the first half of the half, and as I hit the course's six-mile mark, I felt fresh and confident. Steady. All good.

But then I heard an engine humming behind me and a voice over a loudspeaker.

"YOU! You need some water? *You . . . Need . . . Some . . . WATER?*"

I looked back and saw that I had a tail: the race ambulance.

My self-fulfilling prophecy arrived in the form of bullhorning EMTs who kicked the piss out of my confidence and downgraded my pace from steady to slow-ass lumpy boy. Once those blue-shirted and goodhearted ego busters spoke up, I knew I was toast. In the back, again. Slower than everybody else, again. A disaster, again. Humiliated, again—just like my days in gym class.

Though I had dabbled in some weekend warrior sports in my twenties, this was the longest test of my endurance up to this point in my life. And in my first test, I debuted as the human caboose. When it hit me that I must have been not just in the back of the pack but the back of the back of the pack, my pace slowed from a first gear to an *is-he-going-in-reverse?* plod.

It grew lonelier and lonelier as the morning waned and the crowd thinned out. I felt defeated, deflated.

I saw nobody near me when I trudged up a quarter-mile hill, the biggest on the course, at about mile eleven. Near the top, a car pulled alongside me.

It was one of my editors, Peter, a fit, slim, healthy man whose reputation at *Men's Health* was that he tried every single tip we printed. Later, he'd nickname me Steaming Bull because of the steam that rose from my body after a cool-temp swim in an outdoor pool in Pennsylvania—and presumably because I resembled an angry animal. I always liked Peter because he was a gentleman—polite even when he needed to be critical, encouraging even when he may have wanted to tell you that you sucked.

Peter had long finished the race—and I'm assuming had even spent a good amount of time eating a banana, laughing with friends, and walking to his car—while I still had two miles to go. He rolled down the passenger-side window.

"Spiker," he said. His eyes agonized over the news he had to break. "I think you missed a turn."

I looked back down the hill to see how far off-course I was (meaning I had missed a turn and now had to make up even more distance), and that's when I saw them ahead of me: the walkers.

I blurted out a phrase that rhymes with "snow truck" and darted down the hill.

First, ambulance surveillance. Now the walkers were smoking me. (I had nothing against those walking a race, of course; I just didn't plan on their autobahn-ing past me on the homestretch.)

Eventually, I passed the walkers and finished. Two of my other coworkers were waiting (and waiting and waiting and waiting) at the end. They, too, had finished long ago, one of them zipping around the course so fast that he probably would have had time to run the loop again. But they stood there and clapped, two hours and thirty-some minutes after the gun had gone off, and told me I'd done a good job.

I, of course, knew that I hadn't.

The next morning, Peter fired off an angry e-mail to the race directors, explaining the cruelty of unclear turns. I had run the hardest race, he said, because of the extra miles and minutes.

Though I blamed nobody except myself for my mistake and pace, I remember Bill and Adam standing there for me and what Peter did—they had my back, even if I was the back. When it was all over, people encouraged me. *That's the longest run you've ever done! Look at all the people who don't do it! Be proud—you can do better next time!* Was this nice? Yes. Did it make me feel better? Not really. I was pissed off at my body and my mind for failing me so miserably. But that was the moment I had a choice, as do all people who suffer some form of humiliating moment: crumple or push on.

Likely in large part to the fact that I worked in an environment with fit folks and because of all the encouragement I received afterward, I decided that I wasn't going to turn into a garlic-bread-loving fool. The following year, I significantly improved my time in the half marathon, finished among other runners rather than at the very back, and for the first time in a long while, dropped my weight to under two hundred pounds.

Now, I admit that none of my humiliating moments have been soul-crushing, probably because I haven't spent all that much time in the grossly overweight category. But having written about weight loss and health over the years and having talked to many folks who have dropped a dramatic number of pounds, I've learned that the embarrassing moment runs as a theme through the arc of the weight-loss story. Some common ones: Too big to fit onto a roller-coaster. Needing to ask for a seat belt extender on an airplane. A father being asked by his toddler if he's pregnant. The experiences are all different, but the effects are all the same. Hurts, stings, zings.

After the initial flush-faced feeling, the choice is: What do you do with that moment?

Do you use it to reinforce what you already think about yourself (i.e., *I'm a mayo-loving sorry excuse for a human being and that's all there is to it!*), or do you use it to energize you into motion to make a change (*Enough!*)? That's a choice driven by emotion, but it's still a choice.

The Difference Between Shame and Humiliation

It wasn't until the early 1990s that psychologists started studying the concept of humiliation. One of the reasons: It was a complex experience that involved relationships between people (the victim, the perpetrator, and the witness or imagined witness), whereas most of the psychological research tended to look more at individual and internal experiences. Linda Hartling, PhD, a researcher who has studied the concept of humiliation as the director of the global network Human Dignity and Humiliation Studies, told me that to understand how to get past humiliating moments, the first thing to do is differentiate between shame and humiliation, two terms that are often used interchangeably. Shame is more of an internal feeling. When people feel shame, they tend to believe they deserve this feeling because they see themselves as unworthy or as having behaved in a way they feel unworthy of their values. Humiliation, on the other hand, can be an internal experience or an external event (or even something brought on by social issues such as poverty). These feelings of humiliation are triggered by an experience of being degraded and devalued in relationship to other people. It's public. "People believe they do not deserve their humiliation," she said. (Until 1757, the word *humiliate* had no negative connotations; it was used as a way for someone to show underlings their place in the social order.) Most scholarly definitions of *humiliation* involve negative themes such as degradation, ridicule, loss of dignity, failure of significance, scorn, and being stigmatized. In fairness, some have pointed out that humiliation might provide some pro-social benefits, citing such concepts as demonstrations of loyalty. (Think of how military training is sometimes portrayed.) Yet, Hartling and her colleagues suggest, the efficacy of humiliation to achieve those benefits is dubious, because it has a tendency to backfire, often leading to negative consequences.

This distinction between shame and humiliation may be one some people don't give much thought. In the locker room, I might be well aware that my hips are toppling over my shorts; and yeah, maybe I ought to opt out of dessert next time; and yeah, maybe I am ashamed of the way I look and what I've eaten to get this way. But for you to sing a little song about my love handles? Screw. Off. (You think this, but not when you're in the actual position of having your love handles sung about; when you're in the moment, you sheepishly take it, ignore it, and then write about it thirty years later.) Shame is internal; humiliation exposes you to the world.

In early studies, Hartling noted that women reported slightly more humiliating experiences than men, perhaps because women traditionally have been evaluated by their appearance. Today, men are facing more of this evaluation, yet they may find it challenging to acknowledge feelings of humiliation, "because admitting to being humiliated is humiliating in itself," Hartling said.

To more clearly understand how hard it is to acknowledge one's humiliation, Hartling said, it is helpful to understand a related experience: the dynamics of social pain, which comes from feeling devalued (or excluded) in relationship to others. Sometimes it involves feeling a loss of status in relationships because we have not achieved some external standard of how we're supposed to look or how we're supposed to perform physically. And by not meeting that standard—even when a standard is unrealistic, unhealthy, and sometimes dehumanizing—feelings of social pain are intensified or perpetuated. The same part of the brain that lights up when you feel physical pain, the anterior cingulate cortex, also lights up during social pain. This was first studied by researcher Naomi Eisenberger, PhD, an associate professor in social psychology at UCLA. In her experiment, participants played a virtual ball-tossing game. When they were excluded from the game, the same parts of the brain that light up when someone experiences physical pain lit up in those who felt rejection during this game. The bigger picture: Pain acts as sort of an alarm system, indicating that something's wrong. This makes sense when it comes to physical pain, but also when it comes to emotional pain. Humiliation triggers social pain. Social pain serves as a signal for us to do something to get out of a threatening relationship, to look for healthier relationships, to ensure the survivability of the individual and the species.

Some research suggests that humiliation inflicts a sense of powerlessness. In reaction, some targets will withdraw and internalize their experience as shame, perceiving the event as their fault. They blame themselves. This reaction can lead the target down a path of social disconnection and depression. One study of more than seven thousand twins found that humiliation was the second most significant predictor of major depression, behind only the loss of an important relationship. Another reaction to humiliation is anger and outrage, which is externalized in acts of retaliation and revenge. This reaction can lead us down a path of aggressive behavior and misguided attempts to reclaim a sense of power and dignity by wielding power over others. (Some scholars have noted a history of humiliation in the lives of individuals who went on to engage in acts of violence, including school shooters.)

But there are constructive responses to humiliation. Men, for example, often use humor to defuse humiliating moments (*Look at me, the dolt!*), deflect conversation, show the world they're not bothered, while women tend to defuse the impact of humiliating experiences by using their social networks to debrief and to repair their sense of worth in connection to others.

In *The Big Guy Blog*, which I write for *Runner's World* magazine, I use both tactics (humor and social networking), mocking my size or noting the irony of having Bow Wow Wow's "I Want Candy" on my running playlist. I make fun of myself—perhaps so others can't, but also because I think humor can show that I own my issues and don't take myself too seriously. But my wife doesn't like it. She thinks that my self-mocking is a cover, that if I continue to barb myself, then there's no way I can change my attitude to become the thinner and leaner version I've always said I've wanted. Her point: Keep saying you're an oaf, and you're an oaf. Start thinking lean and strong, and that's what you'll be.

I've always argued that there is value in using humor as my baggy sweater, to cover up what's really underneath. In a story for *American Scholar* magazine, neuroscientist Richard Restak, MD, explained that there are several theories for how humor works. One is the tension-release theory, in which tension counterbalances some assumptions we may have about a situation. Another is the superiority theory, which emphasizes how we use humor to focus on a person's mistakes. Restak wrote that this theory explains so-called hostile jokes—jokes that make us feel better about ourselves because they largely put down others. But in my case, and in the case of others who use self-deprecating humor, it's about putting down ourselves, perhaps as a way of letting others connect to us, to let people know that we share similar experiences—experiences that feel so unique and isolated but are actually far from it. (Schools and gym classes, Hartling noted, "are sadly too often humiliation factories.")

The value of using that deflection may actually lie in this juxtaposition: When we feel bad about ourselves, the self-deprecating humor actually acts as some sort of boost. One University of New Mexico study published in *Evolutionary Psychology* looked at the use of this kind of humor. Unsurprisingly, researchers found that men used the tactic more than women. In one part of the experiment, participants listened to audio recordings of people using different types of humor; the participants were later asked to rate the attractiveness of those telling the stories. Researchers concluded that high-status men who used self-deprecating humor increased their long-term attractiveness. Attractiveness did not change for those men labeled as low-status (researchers theorized that high-status people could afford to use humor, seemingly because they had other qualities that would be deemed attractive by others). It should be noted that researchers did not examine the correlation between attractiveness and type of humor used by wide-hipped men.

Who Owns the Power of the Moment?

I asked Hartling what the deciding factor was that made one person respond to a humiliating experience with depression, aggression, or other negative emotions while another person responded with energy, purpose, or a drive to change. Research shows that people tend to fall in the first category.

"If people are connected to a community or just in an open and supportive relationship," Hartling said, "chances are that they'll head in a constructive direction and toward a healthy response." In fact, in one of her recent research papers, Eisenberger wrote that this kind of social pain does have value. Although the experiences of social pain are distressing and hurtful, she wrote, they can serve a valuable function, "namely, to ensure the maintenance of close social ties." That is when we have a negative reaction to humiliating experience, the potential exists for us to make or enhance our social connections as our loved ones show empathy and support.

I've seen this firsthand—the power of the group to steer someone either in the right direction or send someone retreating tongue-first into a pint of Cherry Garcia ice cream. That's because this whole battle with weight isn't about shifting responsibility to others, but rather figuring out how to harness the power of others to help you find your own way. I've felt it work both ways—not in pop-your-pants kind of humiliating moments, but stinging ones nonetheless.

When I worked at *Men's Health*, a group of us signed up to run an adventure race, a half-day event that required the group to move as a team, swimming, running, mountain biking, canoeing, and climbing mountains. I joined a team of three other men and one woman. The three guys were all studs—fast, athletic, cardiovascular beasts who could walk faster than I could run—and they'd be able to crush the course. The woman and I were on similar ground when it came to speed. I had worried about holding them back, but they assured me it was all for the fun, the adventure, and hey, we'd have a good time. I loved that they let me on their team (even though I wasn't their athletic peer) because I wanted the adventure of the adventure.

Early on in the race, at a point when two of us rode mountain bikes for three miles while the other three ran, I was rolling down a slight downhill, picking up speed, when I lost control and hit the ground. When I got up, I looked at my bike.

I had just completed the most cliché act that a big man can do. I had broken the seat.

Sheared that sucker right off the stem. There was no way to fix it on the spot, or even at the next checkpoint.

So I rode to the next stop, about a mile and a half away, standing up.

On the next leg, we all had to ride bikes (ten or twelve miles), and I knew I would not be able to ride the whole way sans seat. I didn't want to bail. I didn't want to let the group down. I didn't want to be the reason we'd have to withdraw—because that, too, would have been cliché. *Of course, fat boy can't finish.*

My teammates laughed, and we debated possible solutions. Right then, another team from the same company passed us and asked what had happened.

"Oh, I've got another seat," one guy said. "Hang on."

Their support vehicle was nearby, and he popped the new seat on, and off we went.

My ass had failed me, but he'd saved it.

We finished the race (albeit toward the back), and I trudged along the best I could with my team. I knew I had slowed them way down, especially on the long stretch of bike trail and the hike up the mountain. Afterward, one of our team members was talking to some of his friends who had competed on another team and had recorded a blazing time. He didn't know I could hear him. He never said my name, but I knew he hated that our time didn't reflect his ability.

"Fucking embarrassing," he said.

Was he right? From his perspective, yes. Had I done anything wrong (besides *break a seat*)? Probably not. Do I wish I could have performed better, been smaller, moved faster? Yes, of course. Did it scar me, having one of my teammates pseudo-trash-talk me to other folks? No, not really. I didn't need to be coddled, and I didn't care all that much about what he said. He was trying to save face with his fit peers, so I got it. But I remember exactly how I felt the second I heard it: My weight (which wasn't even all that high at the time) was no longer about me. It was affecting others. And how others perceive us absolutely shapes how we feel about ourselves and the subsequent actions we take.

Hartling made the point that these humiliating moments—even if they last for only a few seconds or minutes—stick for a long time, and they're some of the freshest and most vivid memories people will ever have, which points to the power of one instance to have lasting effects. For example, I took a look at an online fitness message board. The topic: "Your Most Humiliating 'Fat' Experience." A sample of what I read:

- "My husband said I should get a bigger swimsuit. I was wondering what he meant and why he said that. He would never really clarify. Finally, he just yelled at me and told me I looked disgusting in my swimsuit." (Multiple people responded: "Why are you with this man?")
- "I was at Wal-Mart once and spotted this really short lady trying very hard to reach the milk stuck all the way at the back of the cooler cabinet. So I offered to get it for her. She said, 'Oh, that would be nice of you, dear, but you should not be bending over like that when you are pregnant.' Needless to say, I am not."

- "I was a junior in high school and prom dress shopping. The saleswoman asked me to leave the store because they didn't make dresses for people my size (I was an 18 then). She wouldn't even let me touch the gowns."
- "I couldn't fit into a roller-coaster seat at Six Flags when I was around 15. It was so humiliating because the workers tried and tried to get the seat to lock. When it didn't work, I had to get up and walk away with everyone staring at me. I remember walking to the nearest food stand and getting a large soda to drink."
- "Growing up, my dad always called me fat boy. When I was in my 20s, he apologized, unprompted, and I am good with that, but I look back at it and I think it was what made me what I was."
- "While out running, I got yelled at by a passing car. 'Keep running, fat ass!'"
- "In middle school I rode a bus that was so overcrowded that we had to sit three to a seat. I got on early enough to sit down first, and when the bus driver told a kid to sit next to me the kid said, 'But there are already three people in that seat.'"
- "In gym class, we had to get weighed in front of everyone and your weight got yelled across the gym to another teacher to calculate our BMI (body mass index). When I stepped on the scale, it said, 'error,' so I was known as 'error' that year."
- "When I realized I would crush my wife if we did it missionary style."
- "Guys chanting, 'Cookie, cookie,' when I ran in gym class."

Of all the posts, I was drawn to two stories in particular. In one, a woman recounted hitting a girl in ninth grade because she was being mean to her. She was sent to the principal's office and told the principal that she was suicidal because she was fat and felt worthless. The principal asked her what she was doing to change that, and the woman said she was walking to school and had lost fifteen pounds. The principal's response: "I don't believe you. I'm sure you splurge on Häagen-Dazs and pizza once in a while."

Then she was suspended.

"Those were the exact words she used, and I never forgot them," the woman wrote, "and I brought it up to her when I was a senior and she denied ever saying it. When you confide in an adult that's supposed to help you and they tell you something like that, it's the kind of thing that you just don't forget."

I was also drawn to the story of another woman. In second grade, a boy named her Jack-o'-Lantern because she was big and round. And in sixth and seventh grade, she arrived to school late and would have to walk into the classroom in front of everyone. "The teenage boys would make noises like I was shaking the earth and whisper loudly, 'BOOOM . . . BOOOOOOM . . . BOOM' every time I took a step."

Some people on the message board explained how those moments crushed them, but some talked about how, while they vividly remembered the embarrassment, they'd moved past it, learning that if you let others control who you are and what you think about yourself, they've won and you've lost. Sometimes it just takes reframing what happened.

Getting Past Our Past

The posts went on and on and on. Vivid memories. Some from a few days ago, some from years ago, but the common theme was clear: Just a few words or actions have the power to stick with you and send you into a decades-long funk about how you look and who you are.

"Kids in general are resilient. It's amazing how much they can bend and flow," said Kathy Kater, a clinical social worker who specializes in body image and weight concerns, especially among children and adolescents. "But we also know that the old saying about sticks and stones really isn't true. In fact, children suffer a great deal, and often permanently, from teasing and harassment and being the victim of various kinds of prejudices. In our culture, there probably isn't any '-ism' more endorsed than size-ism, than weight-ism. When children are teased for their size and shape, it's not an isolated thing. It's something that they know has an entire culture behind it."

Kater told me that too often our messages to children are part of the problem. If a child gets big, we start talking about diets and weight and all the things we talk about as adults, but "the research is pretty clear on this," she said. "In many ways, the more people worry about fatness and weight and eat in ways designed to control weight, the less likely they'll be able to sustain a healthy weight over time." The same holds true for bodily dissatisfaction: The more dissatisfied kids are with their bodies, the less likely they'll be able to eat healthily and the more likely they will be to gain weight. This creates that long-term self-fulfilling cycle and the traumatizing effect of never quite feeling good enough.

"Most of my work in thirty-five years has been with adults,"

Kater said. "I see the effects of what happened when they were ten, when they were eight. And body shame is the hardest thing to overcome. People can learn to do the healthy behaviors—not skipping meals, eating well, staying active—but if they are not able to learn to reconnect with and truly care about their bodies, they are not going to be able to maintain those positive behaviours over time."

Part of the problem is the bias we have about weight, she said. If someone tries hard and gets a D in math class, we chalk it up to "He's just not good at math, ha ha ha." But if the same happens in gym class, we say, "That's something you should be able to control." Kater said that until we can collectively start seeing that healthy people come in different shapes and sizes, larger kids will continue to be stigmatized, demoralized, and ultimately less able to make positive choices.

So while we can't control how others think of us or what they say, we can control our response: Do we use the humiliating experience as a reason to retreat from the world, or do we use it as some form of alarm—that maybe something is wrong and we should do something about it? It's hard to choose the latter, because the kids who yell, "BOOM, BOOM, BOOM," are the ones in the wrong, so we don't want them to have any influence on decisions we make or even give them credit for inspiring change. Yet if we can somehow take away their surface-level power, their ability to make us feel bad, and make them realize that we're the ones with the power, we will have flipped the switch—and redistributed the power from the a-holes to ourselves.

On the day of our final basketball game in eighth grade (on the team I made only because I was student government president), we held a pep rally in front of the school. One of the captains assigned us all nicknames. As the least talented player on the team, I was one of the three members of the "Airball Express." I laughed off the distinction—maybe because I wasn't singled out as the only member, or maybe because I had a good group of friends in school, or maybe because I was the resident multiplication tables ass-kicker and I could exert my testosterone and pump up my stats in math class with rapid-fire answers in one-on-one battles: *21, 42, 66, 9, 45, 18, 81, 36, 32 . . .*

Near the end of the pep rally, the captain told the school to come out to the final game (a) because it was the final game and (b) "to watch Ted score his first points of the season."

It was all true. We had been through maybe ten or twelve games; I saw playing time in nearly all of them because our coach was good about giving all the kids a chance to play. But I never scored, and I was the only one on the team who hadn't. I didn't shoot all that often, probably because I shied away from the ball (better not to fail, right?).

This last game, though, I embraced my distinction as the underdog.

In the pregame meeting, when our coach went over starting lineups, I was sure I'd get the nod. I didn't, but he did tell the team, "Let's get Ted a score."

I came into the game in the second quarter and immediately took a shot.

Whistle. Foul. Two free throws.

So this is how it ends, I figured. Nail a couple of free throws and get the zero off my name.

I missed the first. Then I missed the second.

When I came out of the game, I sat at the end of the bench

trying to hide my tears. Humiliated about my public failure, again. Nice try, but you still suck.

In the fourth quarter, I reentered the game. With about two minutes left, I caught a pass to the left of the free-throw line and took a jump shot.

Swish.

Two points. For the entire season.

In my mind, the crowd erupted. Inside, I did.

I remember doing a very small and low-key fist pump to the ceiling after the shot, but reports after the game were that in the moment after the shot went in, it was the highest anyone had ever seen me jump.

Coach took a time-out, and I was prepared to be showered with verbal ticker tape when I returned to the bench. Instead, Coach huddled everyone up and started talking end-of-game strategy. In the middle of his instructions, he turned to me, subdued, and said, "Nice shot, Ted." He then continued with what we had to do to close out the game.

At the time, I wanted more, craved more, wanted acknowledgment from my coach that the slightly plump eighth-grader who got a D in gym class had hit a clutch shot.

Looking back, I see that Coach gave me exactly what I wanted: to be treated like the rest of the team and not—as I was told—that I was lucky to even be on it.

PART 2

Down Size: Getting Going

Truth: Data Is Only a Fraction About Numbers

On one assignment a few years ago, a camera crew filmed me doing a workout. When I saw the outtakes, I cowered—my butt looked like a basketball arena. I confessed to the producer, who knew my history and struggles, that I couldn't believe my gluteus extended beyond my maximus.

"But you own it and have fun with it," he said. "So I think it's all good."

I said, "Yeah," while noticing he didn't tell me it didn't look that big.

I have tried to own my size and shape. I haven't liked it, of course, but I've rarely wallowed. Frustrated? Yes. Used self-directed barbs as a coping mechanism? All the time. But pitied myself? No. Blamed others? Not even my run-another-lap gym teacher. Those methods of dealing with body issues have their risks, including: the outside voices that help shape your perception of yourself. I don't remember being called too many blubber-centric names growing up, but these barbs from my college years stick out:

- A roommate nicknamed me Hoover for the speed with which I ate. Once, during a meal at Wendy's, he broke down the nickname like a color commentator as he analyzed my eating form. I kept my chin hovering as low to the plate as possible, he said, to minimize the distance from plate to mouth. (This is the same roommate who showered with his pet rats.)
- Some friends told me that the only reason I was effective in our pick-up basketball games was because I played "big-butt defense." That is, I used my backside like a front-end loader and moved people to places I wanted them to go.
- During my time working at the college newspaper, one guy would yell, "Dog pile!" or find some other physical way to counteract the stress of putting the paper out, whether it was wrestling or playing office basketball with a tennis ball and a *Planet of the Apes* trash can. When one buddy described my wrestling prowess, he said, "Spiker is tough to bring down because of his low center of gravity . . . and those childbearing hips."

I couldn't, and didn't, argue with any of the assessments, and they didn't even bother me all that much (though an argument can be made that my remembering them so vividly may indicate otherwise). All in fun. Ha ha ha. Spiker has a big butt. So what? It is what it is. But as weight (and sensitivity) increases, we don't want to know how others might see us. So we avoid mirrors. We hate having pictures taken. We stick the scale in the linen closet underneath the set of towels that no one uses and on a shelf along with the Benadryl from 1996. We don't *want* an assessment. Better just to eat the ice-cream sandwich than—cue Beethoven's Fifth—know the truth.

We hide.

The day in 2007 when I stepped on the scale and saw 279 pounds, I knew I probably could have prevented that number from going so high if I had just taken three seconds and weighed myself months earlier. If I had faced up to those three digits, I could at least have prevented some of that weight gain (even though it needs to be said that weight isn't the only number we should use to judge our health).

That stage—the bridge from avoiding the facts to gathering the facts—serves as a crucial step in going from problem to solution. The message that we have to tell ourselves: Stop avoiding and start asking, "What in the name of cheesy chips are we dealing with here?"

There are two ways to do it: One is the literal look in the mirror. That's where we come to grips with our shape, with where we store fat, with how we look. The danger is that our perceptions and our judgments are way harsher than reality. Too often we see all our flaws (or what we perceive as flaws) and beat ourselves up about them. The other way to do it is to be even more literal—get a wide range of assessments from various points of data, be it the scale or a blood test or any number of markers. Many of us tend to avoid those numbers for the same reason we avoid mirrors. We know we're not going to like what we see, even though that hard data can serve as the impetus for change.

Making that change takes some acknowledgment of both methods of assessment—some subjective and some objective. Is any one piece the symbol for the whole problem? Probably not. But collecting all the data serves as a starting point for any project. It's what we do in almost any other facet of our lives: At work, we collect data before we can make changes. At home, we need to hear both sides of the story, from sibling one and sibling two, before figuring out who gets punished and how. We use that information to establish the baseline, to identify problems, to see the whole picture, then to come up with solutions. Somehow in the weight-loss game, we don't approach things the same way. Why? Because it hurts too damn much to step on the scale or see the blood work or see a photo in which you're wider than everyone else. So we ignore, and we resist, and we feel guilty for ignoring and resisting, so we head to the pantry for a sleeve of Nutter Butters. To start the process honestly means coming clean with the two-pronged inspection: the subjective and objective assessments. Here are mine.

Subjective: Muscles in spots, but shaped with wide hips and a bulbous butt.

Objective:

Height: 6'2"
Maximum Weight: 279
Weight Tracker:
End of college, 1990: 180
1993: 231
1994: 190
1998: 200
2000: 222
2001: 195
2006: 229

2007: 279
2008: 250ish
2010: 235ish
2011, early: 262
2011, late: 240
2012: 225
2013: 220
2014: 200ish

Blood Tests: Thankfully, I've always had strong numbers, such as cholesterol (under 200 for total cholesterol) and blood pressure (crept a little high when I weighed the most, but most times it measures normally, in the 115/75 range). When I weighed in the 260 range, I had borderline high blood sugar, but lowered it by the next year. By all other tangible tests, other than the scale, I've always been healthy. Here, some would use the label "healthy obese," a state in which one's weight is higher than it should be, but there are no signs of organ damage or issues involving any of the blood-related factors associated with obesity. One study of twins (one who was obese and one who wasn't) published in the journal *Diabetologia* explained the reason: The fat cells in the healthy obese stay near the skin, while the fat in people who suffer from related health problems get sent to the organs, damaging them in the process.

Maximum Waist Size (Measured in Pants Size): 48. (Disclaimer: My waist did not need the size-48 pants, but that was the size I needed to get over my hips and butt.) I bought size 48s the day after I weighed in at 279. When I dropped down to a size 40, my waist measured about a 36, but I couldn't fit size-36 pants over my lower body. This, healthwise, is a good thing, because it indicates that my fat is not the visceral, damaging kind, but the kind farthest away from my organs.

Best Pair of Pants I Ever Wore: Back when I weighed in the low 200s and right after my wife had our twin boys, I looked at a pair of jeans my wife had worn right after her pregnancy. As far as I could tell, they looked gender-neutral in color, stitching, and in most other ways—with one exception: They were cut to fit a woman—that is, they were smaller in the waist and roomier below it. To this day, I can't tell you what possessed me to slip on her postpregnancy pants, but I did. And they fit. So I stole them. And wore them. In public. Never had a pair of pants fit as well as they did.

Objective Data:
Find and Reach Small Goals

Anyone wanting to make changes needs to gather and confront at least some of this kind of objective data. While the initial reaction to data may come in the form of depression, stress, or *Did he just admit to wearing women's pants?*, such data are crucial to weight-loss success because they provide the framework for constructing reasonable goals. Michael Roizen, MD, whom I've worked with for years on the *YOU: The Owner's Manual* series of books, told me, "You have to measure something that gets people to feel success." The objective standards may include weight, waist size, blood pressure, cholesterol, and fasting blood sugar. The point is to establish some kind of baseline against which you can track data, and use incremental goals to keep you moving forward.

Roizen remembers one couple who came in to see him—the man wanting an overall wellness check, the wife watching over. Roizen asked the man if he could walk up two flights of stairs without getting out of breath, and the man answered, "Sure." The wife rolled her eyes and said, "Honey, the last time you walked two flights of stairs, Eisenhower was president." Roizen likes the stairs test because it gives him a quick assessment of heart health, but it also gave the man a test he could do at home to see how he was progressing—his perceived level of being out of breath versus the numbers of steps he'd climbed. Here, process trumps goal.

Another time, a patient e-mailed Roizen asking how in the world she was supposed to walk ten thousand steps a day (Roizen's prescription when coaching people trying to lose weight) when she was in a wheelchair for a variety of ailments. So Roizen asked her if she walked at all. She said, yes, to the bathroom. He asked her, "If I send you a pedometer, will you count your daily steps?" She did, and e-mailed him the answer: "Sixty-four."

Roizen wrote back, telling her that all he wanted her to do was increase the number of steps she took every day. It didn't matter by how many, just that there was an increase. That's what she did, and she never had a day when she didn't increase her steps from the previous day. Two years ago, she was able to get rid of her wheelchair, and one year ago, she was able to get rid of her walker. She lost weight and got healthier, and Roizen said a big factor in this was that she had that baseline against which to measure some kind of goal. "You can't deny asthma, but there's a huge amount of denial with obesity," Roizen said. "I don't think scaring motivates people to stay on a program. What motivates them is success and rewards." Which is why, Roizen said, objective data

matter—and are a crucial step toward changing habits and, ultimately, bodies. They're important also because they're part of the
way we view process over end goals: Focus on the collection and
tracking of some kind of number.

I've seen it work in so many of the people I've talked to who
have lost weight: They used some kind of data point to drive them
to their goals. Just the act of recording a number, and watching it
change, served as the key part of the solution. Research suggests
that the kind of data doesn't even matter; it's the act of choosing a
number, tracking the number, then using that number to inspire
behaviors that does. The most traditional piece of data, of course,
is the number on the scale: it's the number that drives so much of
our angst. There's evidence that tracking weight can work.
Weighing oneself daily is one of the common characteristics of
people on the National Weight Control Registry who have maintained a one-hundred-pound weight loss. The study detailing
these results showed that more frequent weighing was associated
with a lower BMI, compared to less frequent weighing. Weight
tracking can have some flaws, especially for people just starting
out. For one, weight fluctuates depending on such factors as water
weight, hormonal cycles, and muscle changes. At least for me,
seeing no change in weight (or worse, upticks) can lead to frustration, which has the effect of pissing you off, which means that
you're more likely to take out your emotions on a bulk bag of
Bugles. I like the scale for monitoring once you've made some
progress, but not so much at the beginning of a weight-loss quest,
because you can see such little movement when you're putting in
such huge efforts in those first couple days and weeks.

The point of self-monitoring, though, isn't to beat yourself up about the number on the scale, or any number, really. It's about having some kind of tangible feedback for the work you're doing, so you can do just as we do with data in other parts of our life—look at it, analyze it, use it to adjust goals, and win the day. So data collection is really just about picking anything that will help keep you on track—whether it's calories per day, or steps walked, miles run, blood pressure lowered, ounces of water consumed, push-ups performed, anything. What number can you use to see if you improve from one day to the next? String enough of those numbers together, and you've got a better chance of seeing the other number, the one on the scale, move where you want it to go.

A review published in the *Journal of the American Dietetic Association* looked at twenty-two studies on self-monitoring. Most of the studies used dietary tracking as the method for self-monitoring, while a handful used body weight and exercise activity. While the review authors noted some study limitations (one being the fact that the studies were based on self-reporting—that is, since the data came from the individual, there was no control over whether they were accurate), they also noted these findings: All studies that focused on dietary self-monitoring (food journals, calorie counting) showed that these had significant associations with weight loss. The more frequently people self-monitored, the better their weight loss, though there was no conclusion about how frequently one should self-monitor for success. Just the act of seeing numbers in some kind of context can help change behavior. A study presented at the Experimental Biology meeting looked at people's ordering habits when menus displayed no calorie information or the amount of walking that would need to be done in order to burn off those calories. The Texas Christian

University researchers found that having such calorie and exercise data on menus led to fewer calories ordered than when two other menus without such data were used.

Some argue that there's no need to track calories or steps or weight if you're eating the right way and moving throughout the day, but for many of us, these provide the tools we need to get going. Self-monitoring seems to be one of the key predictors of successful behavior change for many people, said Angela Kong, PhD, a postdoctoral fellow at the University of Illinois at Chicago who has studied the subject. It may help people be more aware of what they are trying to change and perhaps offer the necessary feedback to achieve those changes, she said.

In addition to self-monitoring, setting shorter-term, definable goals can help. So saying you want to eat more vegetables might not be as effective as saying you want to aim for two servings of vegetables for dinner every night. Simply put, if you can define the behavior, you're more likely to achieve it.

Derek Daniels, PhD, associate professor of psychology and director of the behavioral neuroscience graduate program at the University at Buffalo, is a data junkie who tracks all his runs via miles and times. When he sees he's plateauing in terms of performance, he uses the data to make adjustments. Though he chalks up his attention to data detail to his scientist personality, he believes that one of the reasons self-monitoring works so well is not only because it helps us feel accountable to our goals, but also because it forces us to pay attention to data that could easily be ignored.

Example: You know you need to lose weight, you eat well most of the time, you go out with your friends, get caught up in the fun of it, and order a plate of food that has more calories than a healthy-weight person would eat in a day. But you rationalize it: *I had fruit this morning. It said "chicken" nachos, and chicken is good for you. It's Friday, and I'm at Friday's—it's meant to be!* But when you're tracking calories and know you have an allotment for the day and the chicken nachos will put you past Friday's count (and Saturday's), you make a different choice. "I think as humans, there are just things that work better when we pay attention to them," Daniels said.

The downside to these types of approaches: It's inconvenient to track every morsel of food—log everything, look up everything, write it down. It takes some doing, and some commitment. Of course technology makes the process easier, especially for exercise, as watches, gadgets, and phones can log and graph all the data (once you enter your vitals in these devices) in whatever form you want, whether it's distance, calories, or speed. The other appeal is that these gadgets and apps mean that you don't have to be sedentary to do self-monitoring, said Brie Turner-McGrievy, PhD, of the University of South Carolina, who studies tech and health. Moving your body actually becomes part of the data collection. Devices such as the FitBit are attached to your body and calculate your movement and steps throughout the day (so it's a pedometer and can collect other data, too). You do the physical work, but it does the data collection.

The process is a little more complicated when it comes to the nutrition aspect. While apps and databases can make logging calories a little more user-friendly, you still have to look up food counts, estimate portion size (unless you're weighing and measuring everything you eat), and log the data. It's not an hours-long task, but it's still a mild annoyance that a lot of people can't sustain for long periods. According to Turner-McGrievy, researchers are now working on nutritional technology that can work more closely with the exercise technology: You take a photo of your food, and when you bite into it, the technology logs the calories—a pedometer for potato skins, if you will. It's still far away from being commercially available (or even close to being accurate). The bigger point is that logging food data—the most influential of all data when it comes to weight loss—puts the onus on the eater; you have to look up, record, and use that data to make changes.

I've tried food journaling several times throughout my own weight-loss efforts, and it worked every time. It helped me stay accountable, and it made me think twice about taking three scoops instead of two. I liked it because I saw results, but I also hated feeling tied to the journal—that I had to log every butter-covered morsel that I ate. I felt tremendously deflated not just when I had to see the calorie counts, but also when I missed my calorie ceiling on a particular day. In the end, I did see the scale numbers move in the right direction, because of two reasons: that accountability to a calorie ceiling and being forced to choose better-for-you foods if I wanted to eat more. (So to save yourself some room, you choose more vegetables and more lean meats and don't blow your day on a few bites of a candy bar.) It teaches you to eat right to stay satisfied. The other way it worked: Once you go through the process of figuring out the calorie count for the foods you make (meaning you plug in certain ingredients, to obtain the calorie count for each), you tend to go back to those foods you already know are healthy because you don't feel like adding up another number. So, to make it easier, you limit your choices. Eventually, you remember how many calories are in a certain food so you won't need to look it up again. And, the hope goes, you'll have taught yourself to eat better and will have made it habit.

The one time I felt that it worked best—and I lost about ten or twelve pounds in a few months using this method—I decided to track my calories, but I made what I thought was an effective adjustment: Instead of having a daily goal, I set a weekly goal of 10,000 calories—the calories I consumed minus the calories I burned (very similar to the Weight Watchers points and bank approach). For the two months that I did it, I loved it, because I had a huge incentive to exercise (it would allow me more food) and I made it a game to see how far under the 10,000-calorie net I could go to give myself some more wiggle room for cheat meals at the end of the week.

The weekly approach worked well for me, because it helped me adjust my eating to my personality. I ate well 90 percent of the time, which eliminated the guilt when I earned some calories to indulge in. It worked much better than a daily goal had, because a daily goal didn't give me much of a buffer. To this day, it is one of my favorite strategies, because it worked for *me*. It may not work for you. The question is: Can you figure out what to monitor and track that fits your personality? Data-driven people may prefer to spreadsheet every bite, while others get sidetracked after three days of trying to count. If you can match your personality to some kind of monitoring system, then you'll likely put yourself in a position to succeed.

Eventually, I gave up counting calories for the reason many people do—it's high-maintenance, and if you can ballpark your calories and learn to eat healthy foods, you don't need to "count." In 2014, I gave my self-monitoring more of a fitness slant. I decided I would track all my exercise with yearly goals. I came up with what I wanted to hit (20,000 push-ups completed, 1,000 miles run, 1,500 miles cycled, 75 miles swum, 1,500 minutes stretching, 30,000 seconds in the plank position, and 75 hours lifting weights), and I entered my numbers into a database, which took about forty-five seconds a day. I like the change from calories to fitness goals because not only was it lower maintenance, but it also hit some other areas—goal setting and focusing on the little steps of the process. That's really the whole point of self-monitoring, whether you apply it to food, activity, blood pressure, or something else.

(Important note about monitoring calories: It's not smart to restrict calories too much, and in my weekly monitoring strategy, there were some days when my net calories were fairly low. It's not smart to take the limbo approach: "How low you can go?" That's because your body does need fuel, and undereating has plenty of problems, too. For me, it was about creating a splurge zone so I could have meatballs and a couple of glasses of wine on a Saturday night without feeling the guilt. I looked at my diet as a total for the week, not a game to see if I could eat as few calories as possible. That wouldn't work, is not smart, and obviously is the foundation for more traditionally defined eating disorders.)

When I used these counting methods, they worked (and research supports that they do for many people). They helped me eat well most of the time and work out consistently. But having success wasn't all about the numbers. The bigger challenge meant dealing with the mirror.

Body Image: The Most Evil Data of All?

After college, Tina Haupert put on weight, mainly due to her desk job and the fact that she prioritized other things over fitness and healthy eating. She had tried to lose weight, but nothing ever stuck. Her turning point came when she saw photos from a New Year's ski trip.

"I was just shocked. I looked horrible, and I said, 'I need to lose weight,'" she told me. "I think it was just pure shock. 'What happened to me? What happened?'"

On the day Tina saw the photo, she knew she didn't need to lose much weight (about twenty-five pounds), but she decided that a quick fix wasn't going to be the answer. "It might sound cheesy, but instead of doing this terrible diet, I almost had this self-love moment. I realized that I didn't take on the weight overnight, so let's think that getting healthy is going to be good for you—and find ways to eat so you enjoy it. The nice and not painful ways to lose weight," she said.

With the self-imposed deadline of her wedding looming, she lost the weight doing it the way that many others do—calorie counting, making small changes over time, setting goals, and scheduling workouts in her calendar and treating them like appointments she couldn't miss. She started a popular blog called *Carrots 'N' Cake* after she lost the weight and found that the accountability for herself and her readers was a huge motivator in maintaining her good health. It was that full-body inspection, not hiding from the image, that really inspired the change.

"Seeing evidence of my weight gain was a huge turning point for me," she said. "I knew my clothes felt tighter, but I just figured they shrunk a little in the dryer or I was bloated from drinking beer or eating nachos. The photos from that ski trip just made it seem so real." She hated the way she looked, especially in comparison to her college friends, who hadn't gained any weight (and seemed to get healthier after college). "Maybe I was comparing myself to them, but I think the contrast of how I looked compared to my friends, who I used to look like, was the nail in the coffin that ultimately got my butt in gear to lose weight."

This is the area of inspection that's so difficult for many people to address—the subjective data: How we look. How we feel. The flaws. The fat. The size. The ubiquitous question of "Which skirt makes my butt look smaller?" (Note: Despite evidence to the contrary, I have not worn skirts.) We can collect all the data we want, but for many of us, those subjective moments and perceptions are the ones that really count, and because they're so subjective, it's hard to argue with them—whether it's through our own voices or those of the people close to us who assure us that the skirt does not, in fact, make our butts look big.

Body image issues, of course, are the subject of many a book, research article, magazine story, and angel-devil conversation in our heads. Research shows that women are subject to more negative effects of body image issues than men—seemingly because of the collective import that we, as a society, place on femininity and appearance. It's not a one-gender issue, though men typically are more successful at either ignoring or de-emphasizing body insecurities than women. Much of the research about men centers on muscle dysmorphia—that is, unrealistic expectations regarding the amount of muscle a man has and the quest to want more and more. Part of the reason men are hard to study is because, unsurprisingly, they don't see that having more muscle is a problem, so they don't request help for it, and also because they're less willing to talk about any psychological issues they have about feeling fat or misshapen. The central question for either gender, though, is why we're so hard on ourselves? Why don't we see our bodies the way others do? As in, it's probably not as bad as you think. Some experts would argue that so many outside pressures—be they from images we see on all our screens or from the desire to get better jobs/partners/opportunities—make it difficult to ease up on ourselves.

Those who study the subject argue that not only have body image issues not improved, but they also may in fact be getting worse. One driving reason for this is the strong influence of the media—the pervasive "thin is better" message that comes from fashion models and in-front-of-the-camera celebs. Though we have examples that counter that message (Lena Dunham of *Girls* fame being one of the strongest examples of an embrace-all-bodies mantra), the overwhelming message, especially to women, is the one we've been hammered with constantly: The smaller you are, the more glamorous you are. "I saw a story out of Sweden where advertising executives were standing outside an eating disorder clinic interviewing people for a modeling career," said J. Kevin Thompson, PhD, a psychology professor at the University of South Florida who studies body image. (A Swedish paper reported that one of the patients whom the talent scouts approached was so sick that she was in a wheelchair.)

Kids from a very young age get the message—through the media, stories, cartoons—that there are certain standards of attractiveness. "When boys and girls, girls especially, don't meet those standards, they feel bad about themselves," said Lora Park, PhD, an associate professor of psychology at the University at Buffalo who works in the realm of self-worth and attractiveness. "It's a cultural phenomenon, this hyperemphasis on physical appearance more so than being a good, decent person."

Another factor for negative body image is that the beauty business is a massive one that sells us on the notion that we need to get fitter, smaller, and better-looking—and plays into our self-loathing.

My self-loathing? Perhaps I'm in denial, but with the exception of the time I stepped on the scale and saw 279, I don't think I loathe all that much. I get frustrated, I regret making some food decisions, I joke about my shape, and I have cringed at many a mirror and photo. Are those forms of self-loathing? Perhaps. But I don't think I've wallowed. Maybe it's because I use those self-directed insults as the guardian to the gate of darkness. If I laugh about it, all's cool. *Dude's got hips, NBD.* Maybe it's because this is part of who I am. What would happen if my body changed? Would I change? What would happen if I no longer had that "extra gland" to use as my foil?

Central to the whole notion of appearance, weight seems to be one of the prime factors, in addition to race and gender, that strongly influences people's perception of us, Park said. In research from Yale University, scientists argued that while some people may say that issues such as poor body image can motivate people to lose weight, "it is more likely that these form barriers to emotion regulation that, for both biological and psychological reasons, lead to increased eating." The same researchers called negative messages about being overweight "relentless." Fascinating note: There's such a thing as phantom fat—the idea works a little like phantom limbs for amputees, in that people who've lost weight still feel fat and see fat in places where it no longer exists, which explains why formerly fat folks have a hard time embracing new bodies and accepting them as fit and healthy.

The tricky part about body image, of course, is that with our obesity epidemic and the percentage of overweight people ever increasing, the goal is the correct one: Many of us who are overweight do need to lose weight for health reasons. For a good number of us, it's not a bad goal to get thinner—unless it strays too far in the other direction. In fact, maybe for some people, there is value in body dissatisfaction, because it can be productive and lead to change.

So how do you teach that, especially to kids, so that body dissatisfaction doesn't lead to extreme measures such as eating disorders? Thompson said, "I don't know that anybody has figured out how to do it. On the other hand, if obese people have a very positive body image, that could be a problem, too, because they might not be motivated to engage in healthier eating and exercise behaviors."

Thompson had to deal with the issue head-on with his own adolescent son, who was overweight. He struggled with how to talk to him, because of the tricky nature of trying to send a healthy message while not being aggressive or overwhelming. On his own, Thompson's son started walking on the treadmill and cutting out some junk food, and he lost the weight. He made little adjustments, and they worked. Thompson said he never really talked about "weight" with his son. The notion of social comparison did its job in a healthy way—the young man was surrounded by thinner friends, was interested in girls, and made a decision to try to improve his body and health. "We never said he had to lose weight," Thompson said. "He just made his mind up."

Thompson said the issues surrounding body image come down to a phrase called "normative discontent," meaning that pretty much everyone is unhappy with some aspect of their appearance—some people only slightly, some people moderately, all the way up to those people who've snuck on opposite-gender jeans. Traditionally, a lot of blame is directed toward those media portrayals. "If you could magically flatten the landscape and have a wide variety of normal-sized women with diversity and various ethnicities and features, it would have to have a positive effect," Thompson said. "One of the primary effects is through social comparison; you could compare yourself to a wider variety of people."

Of course, it's not easy to change self-perception, Thompson said—and it's not always healthy to automatically have positive self-perception if there are serious health problems that need to be addressed. One of the first things he teaches people is to redistribute the self-image pie. "If appearance is ninety percent of your self-image, then you're not going to be happy most of the time," he said. So what he asks patients to do is list all the things that make up who they are, to try to put appearance in a better context. This can work because so many of us who are influenced by body image issues are simply overwhelmed by them. We can't go a day without thinking about being unhappy with some aspect of our bodies. "We try to get people who primarily think about appearance to think that maybe forty percent or twenty-five percent is appearance and the rest is being a good friend, or a trusted family member, or what you do at work, or your religion, and try to make appearance a reasonable percentage of someone's life," Thompson said. "Then you can try to be reasonable about expectations. Somewhere along that continuum, you can ask, 'What would be the change in percentages that would be good enough? Where you can say I feel a lot better?'" One way to do this, Thompson said, is to literally draw a circle and create slices, or percentages of a pie, that currently represent how you view different aspects of who you are—appearance, friends, career, family, etc. Then draw another circle that represents what you think might be a healthier division of that pie.

One of the answers comes in the form of a full-on, head-on, no-hiding assessment of where you are, not subjectively (in front of the mirror), but regarding the objective data. What is your entire body, and health, story? As a professor who teaches writing, I spend a lot of time critiquing students' work. Sometimes I'll ask for excerpts from an early story draft. I can offer feedback on this, but only a little. Why? Because I need to see the whole story. I need to see how the pieces fit together. I need the context. And when I see that, then I can assess the entire picture (what works, what doesn't) and then offer solutions on how to fix it. That strikes me as one way to approach making bodily changes. Our image, what we see in the mirror, serves as only an excerpt. Once we get the whole story—one that includes self-perception and weight and blood pressure and cholesterol levels and data like that—then we can stop beating ourselves up about having a body we don't like and actually move forward to figure out ways to change our shape, our self-image, and the real data that actually matter.

Thompson's notion of creating a pie makes sense. My fatty hips have preoccupied my mind so many times. They cross my mind when I walk, when I stand up in front of my classes, when I run, when I take a shower. But if you asked the logical side of me to write down all the sides of me as a person that were even semi-important, those hips wouldn't make the list. How, in logical terms, can love handles compete with what I try to do as a father, husband, teacher? But therein lies the struggle: I *know* they don't matter, but that doesn't stop me from feeling that they do.

Redefining your body image is a tough task, no doubt—when

so much of your life revolves around the vessel in which you're carried, how do you de-emphasize the role that body shape and size play? Some would say that there are tangible strategies to help you do that (such as not weighing yourself so often, so that you don't wrap yourself too much into one number), and some would say that making sure you emphasize your social connections helps you change your emphasis on your body. "When you make self-esteem your goal, you're more likely to be vulnerable to depression, more anxious about successes and failures," Park told me. "One solution is to make a shift in thinking about how you can focus on your connection with others, doing activities with other people, helping people, doing something that's larger than yourself. You'll feel less stuck, less concerned about what body image does for your ego. It changes your mind-set."

When you can focus your conversations and thoughts on family, friends, ideas, and dreams, you start to see yourself in the big picture, rather than just being big in a picture.

Redefine Data: The Skill of Feel

Some ten years ago I had an assignment for *Outside* magazine: to write a fitness story about the concept of play. That is, can we move from fitness being about sets and reps, programs and rules, and a chore we have to do, to it being about getting outside, throwing a ball, and exploring? Fitness for fun. Fitness because it feels good to roam and run and play. Fitness because this is what our bodies are meant to do. During the course of reporting that story, one of my sources told me, "You have to talk to Doug Newburg."

Doug Newburg, PhD, a sports psychologist who played basketball at the University of Virginia and later spent his career studying the patterns of elite performers (not just athletes, but also musicians, businesspeople, surgeons), hadn't had the media exposure of more pop sports psychologists. During our talk, he told me about the concept of play and why much of what we do in mainstream sports psychology won't work. Along the way, he sent me a few follow-up e-mails, talking about his work and concepts. When the story came out—and our hour-long interview ended up being boiled down to a sound bite—Newburg wasn't happy. He wrote:

> Saw the Play article in *Outside*. I feel like I completely wasted your time given the one line that actually made it into the article. This of course was absolutely what I expected after talking to the fact checkers, but it really leaves me confused about the process. As I told you when we talked, this is what ALWAYS happens. Anyway, pretty clear to me that doing interviews like this are not worth anybody's time as far as an article is concerned.

After I explained a bit about the process, Newburg wrote back, and we started an e-mail relationship in which we talked about this concept of play—but more important, about his main work involving "feel."

This is the concept that always trips up the media but resonates with every single person he's ever worked with. Newburg has asked the following question to every one of the more than five hundred elite performers he's ever interviewed: "Does how you feel affect the way that you perform?" The answer, 100 percent of the time, is: "Yes, of course." What people don't get is that "feel" is not "feelings." Feel is not about being happy, sad, angry, or any other way we like to define feelings. Feel is different.

Newburg has described it using basketball. "When somebody misses a shot, if it scares them because it affects someone's approval, that is a feeling. If they miss a shot and can feel how it left their hand, they can practice it and correct it." The truth is, "feel" is incredibly hard to define—which is why Newburg ran into so many roadblocks when dealing with media about his work.

Yet we know feel.

Newburg would argue that *these* are the data that matter, the data we can't quantify but that inform all our actions. How we feel when we eat healthy versus how we feel after a pond-size bowl of pasta. How we feel after we go for a run, not how fast or far it was. How we feel when we go dancing. How we feel when we're doing what we love with the people we love: boogie-boarding with your kids, riding a horse, taking a walk with a close friend. None of that has to do with traditional data points—numbers, facts, milestones. It has to do with what you want your life to feel like, and Newburg, I suspect, would ask, how can you measure that in a food journal? Instead, shouldn't we be collecting a different kind of data?

For some people, that sounds sort of psycho-squishy, and that's why he's met with some resistance when discussing this concept. With "feel," there's nothing tangible to wrap your head around—no traditional data point that can prove that you've lost weight, or gotten faster, or gone longer. I remember one time, when I was bitching to Newburg about my slow, sorry-ass times on my run, he asked, "Why do you care?" What did it matter what my times were? I was running, he said, for different reasons, and if I liked the way I felt while I ran or after I'd run, why was I letting a number on a watch change the way I felt during the process? For a few years, Newburg moved to the town where I live, and we had many a discussion about how his concept played out in real life. He told me the story of a junior hockey goalie, maybe seventeen or eighteen, who played elite-level hockey. The young man was feeling the pressure that comes from being a top-tier athlete, and his game was stinking up. He wasn't performing the way he used to. When Newburg worked with the teen, he asked him lots of questions—he never tells people what to do; he asks questions to let them figure it out. Through that process, it came out that the goalie played his best when he thought of himself as a monster—scooping up pucks, standing confident in the net, looking intimidating to opponents. So Newburg asked him again, "Why not think of that when you're playing?" And it worked. It gave the goalie permission to stop getting wrapped up in the pressure and the stats and the idea that he'd better win. It helped him return to what made him successful in the first place. It was about what felt right.

The goalie later sent Newburg this message:

> i dunno if u saw but we got bombed on the weekend.
> destroyed. and i actually felt the same ive felt like all along,
> but its not easy like when the coach starts pointing fingers a
> little and kinda suggests u can play better and its also not
> easy to get scored on like that. So we had a game on
> wednesday and before the game my mind was kinda goin all
> over the place thinkin of things i needed to do and how i
> should be thinking and feeling and i kinda realized like shit
> this isnt good, i shouldnt be having all these things to think

about. So before i went out i was just like fuck it, screw the
stats, screw the attitude that we have to win this one and
that i have to play good. im just gonna go out and love what
im doing and not worry about those things which i did and i
felt the best ive felt in a while. I really pulled off a doug
newburg performance tonight.

Newburg did the same thing with a top college golfer who
was having trouble with her swing. She was thinking too much
and performing poorly on chips to the green. Newburg had an
idea. He stepped about ten feet in front of the golfer and said,
"Hit the ball over my head." The golfer didn't want to, fearing
she'd plunk him in the face. "Don't worry about me. Just hit the
ball over my head." After one timid swing, she took another and
put the ball right on the green. Newburg made his point: Stop
thinking so much that your hand has to be here, your hip there;
that you have to twist this, put this much English on it, whatever
the finer points of mechanics might dictate. Instead, get more in
touch with what you *feel* you need to do to avoid knocking your
coach's four front teeth out of his mouth. Does that mean you
should never use data? Of course not. Newburg's point is that we
have to redefine what data are: Data aren't only quantifiable numbers, stats, graphs, charts, and patterns (though these all have
their place). There are powerful data in feel—if you can be open
to them.

One of the stumbling points, Newburg would argue, is that
we too often let environment and what we suspect other people
think about us get in the way of what we want to do. This applies
to any of us who has struggled with weight loss, not just the elite
performers he's worked with and interviewed.

"I have no problem getting people to do what they need to do as long as they have realized that what they are doing isn't working," he said. "And instead of justifying why they aren't taking care of themselves, why they aren't motivated, they simply say, 'How do I want to feel every day? How do I get there?' They actually pay attention to how they experience themselves and the world around them."

When I was training for my first marathon, I had many discussions with Newburg about my performance and the pressure I felt to perform—which were both actually issues about my body, my feeling that it was bigger than the bodies of most runners and that I'd have a harder time running because of my size. As I was preparing, I often grappled not with my desire to get faster and not embarrass myself, but with my frustrations for not being able to do so. As he's known to do, Newburg sent me a long e-mail, but one that absolutely applies to anyone who's had to deal with weight issues:

> When someone tells you to gut it out, to get off the couch, to not feel what you feel, they are telling you they know better and are therefore better than you. They are judging you. You used the word goals often yesterday. What I am saying is that these "goals" are only good if they fulfill what the subconscious wants, but the problem is that goals are conscious and are often disconnected from the 80% of our brain that is subconscious. The only thing that matters is are we getting closer to connecting with others or moving us closer to that transcendence or resonance[?] What I am arguing is that people don't understand this yet. It is the reason why we do things that is not understood. I don't care if someone reaches their goals if they don't do it in a way that fulfills the subconscious need.

Why? Because most people's goals will allow them to get
2/3 of the way there, but then that same way of getting
where they want to go will prevent them from getting all the
way there. And when we get as far as we can, but can go no
further, the judgment overwhelms the process. And the
judgment of other people, people we either value or give
elevated status to in our lives like experts is the main
obstacle every person I ever work with is confronted with. It
prevents the connection to the thing we're doing and the
performances that would connect us in the ways we want to
connect with others. In other words, it is not understood
that the subconscious is driving the bus. As a result,
expertise on almost everything is about the conscious mind,
the part of the brain that only does 20% of the work. People
who get this, who listen to their subconscious, who "feel"
are more likely to get what they really like and want.

The thing about feel, Newburg said, is that it's not as psycho-
soft as it seems. These are the fundamental feel factors:

1. Feel affects how you perform.
2. Feel is a skill.
3. Feel is data.
4. Feel is a primary motivator.
5. Feel is a reward.
6. How you feel is your responsibility.

To develop feel as a skill, Newburg said, takes paying attention and getting past our normal routines. So maybe it means
running without a watch and just taking note of what course,
what conditions, what pace, feels good—without trying to latch

on to some particular time. With eating, it takes paying attention to how you feel not just during a meal (where, yes, some nastily delicious foods may feel good), but also immediately after and for the rest of the day. Ultimately, it means climbing out of the ruts you're in that aren't getting you where you want to go. If what you're doing isn't working, even if you think it should be, it takes some action on your part to find something that feels and works better. This, Newburg said, is what will lead to deeper motivation, which I'll cover in the next chapter.

I asked him about my Ironman—about how my non-triathlete body would be able to handle the challenges, and what I needed to do to make sure I finished under the seventeen-hour time limit and to avoid both the failure of not reaching my goal and, worse, the public embarrassment for not being able to do so.

"There's a good chance—and I'm not trying to be a dick about it—that it's not going to happen," he told me.

His words stung. I thought friends were supposed to say, "Of course you're going to do it. I believe in you," but he wasn't judging. He was just talking—explaining that just because you set a goal, it doesn't mean everything will fall into place and it will happen. After all, this was probably a little bit beyond my capabilities. Yes, I had made the commitment. Yes, I was training. And yes, I was going to give it a go. None of those things guaranteed results. I still needed to complete my training, and I could get hurt. There was no telling whether I'd get halfway through the bike portion; my knees or back or lungs would hurt and I'd say, "Screw it. I'd rather have a burger." Newburg suspects that my writing about my training on my blog, though it keeps me motivated, contributes to the feeling that I'll let someone down if I fail.

After we got off the phone, he thought about my quest a little more, and perhaps regretted saying there was a good possibility I would fail, so he wrote this:

BUT your entire mission has been about this—to do things you don't think you can do, to prove yourself to others and to yourself, and the doubt and fear that come not from failing to finish, but the belief that somehow you've let other people down. Whether or not you finish is irrelevant to the bigger issue. How you finish matters. Why you finish matters. If finishing is all that matters, if winning is all that matters, then Lance Armstrong would still be a hero. I think you've found a healthy way of doing this that works for you, that sometimes you lose sight of, but then it re-reveals itself to you and you listen to your own body and soul. If you are not being you or a better you, there is no point in trying. Your way leads to a better you. The ONLY thing you want to do is identify and remove the unhealthy tension from your process.

It's easy to turn these things into the pursuit of bliss points, momentary highs that fade, that you have to create over and over again. Those lead you nowhere unless they add up to the experience of transcendence, the connection to other people AND the thing you are doing AND yourself. Choose resonance and transcendence and connection and you'll be fine. You will find out how good you can be at the thing you are doing, but you will also find how good you are as a person, deep inside, and share it with the rest of the world. Don't belittle it by judging yourself by whether or not you finish. If you finished and everyone thought you were a prick or cheated or simply didn't care about you, what you'd find is just hollow sickening emptiness.

During our conversation, Newburg said something that made me relax—and sort of feel like I needed to stop worrying about the end point and what others thought about me—and stop getting wrapped up in the numbers, but start embracing the ups and downs of the journey itself.

"No one is walking around thinking about you," he said. "Maybe people [who read your blog] say, 'That's great; he motivates me.' But then they forget about you until you write something else." And that's when I got it: I had to let go of any pressures I thought were being put on me. The reality is that there really weren't any. "As long as you make an honest effort, and are honest with your audience, you've established those relationships, and they're going to be cheering you on no matter what happens. And in the end, that's what the subconscious is after."

I suspect he might add that there's no so-called scientific data point in the world that can measure that.

Truth: Mojo Is Manufacturable

When Dr. Oz hustled down the stairs to his basement basketball court, it was immediately clear that he was taunting me—not with his words, but with his uniform. He was wearing the same red threads he had donned for his appearance in the 2010 NBA All-Star Celebrity game. Message: He can ball.

He tried to play it off, telling me that he knew my capabilities and that he needed some ammo in the form of intimidation. He leaned into me and told me (in a much saltier way than I'm about to describe) that it wasn't very gentlemanly of him to wear the All-Star getup, "But I knew you'd appreciate it."

What I did appreciate was that in at least one way, we're similar. His uniform sports the number 11—the same number I wore on my eighth-grade basketball uniform.

I had gone to his place to play a game of one-on-one with America's doctor (for a media assignment that never panned out). My mission was twofold: one, to see what I could learn about him, about health, and about competition; and two, to win.

This game pitted Dr. Mehmet Oz, renowned heart surgeon/

Emmy Award–winning TV host/healthiest man alive vs. Schlub with a curb-height vertical jump. Knowing me and my body shape, he had to know my intended tactic: to use my backside to make room and get some easy buckets. So I asked him if he could share a few secrets about how he planned to play me.

"I go to my left much better than you would think. Surgery trains you to be ambidextrous," he said. "I don't shoot very well. For the amount I play, I should be a much better shot. I do hustle. I think that I play cleanly, but you never know."

What I did know is that Oz—who runs, practices yoga, does strength exercises, and once banged out twenty-plus pull-ups on *The Oprah Winfrey Show*—also loves hoops and all kinds of other team sports. (He played water polo and football at Harvard.) So I knew that he was way more athletic than I was, but I hoped that my size would counteract skill. What I failed to anticipate was that he had no intention of losing—especially to me.

"For me, competitive sports are magical," he said. "It's not just about what you can do. It's about how you read the person opposite you."

After he rattled off the house rules (to a score of 11 by ones; make it, take it; no blood, no foul), Oz came out firing—trying to steal on every dribble, grabbing every offensive rebound, going for his favorite shot (a midrange jumper to the left of the free-throw line). His promise ("I do hustle") was an understatement.

Within the first ten seconds, I knew I was doomed—not only because he's a better player, but also because of his intensity.

Oz was up 2–1 when he stole the ball, stepped back, and hit another jumper. I tried to go inside, but he used both hands—as he said he would—to knock my dribble off so I couldn't get low. Within minutes, he was the syrup, I was the pancake, and he smothered me from every direction. I found myself down 5–1 after he chased his own rebound and scored. That's when he started taunting and toying with me. He knew he had me—and this is key—without ever stepping into you-suck territory.

"Let me check his pulse," Oz joked to the camera crew.

"I think we need a video time-out," I wheezed.

His aggressiveness startled me, but it shouldn't have. He ran, he chased, he hustled, he contested everything I tried to do—because he plays hoops the way I expected him to after years of knowing him. Driven, competitive, encouraging, fun—he was beating me by using both body and mind.

I missed a baby hook (my go-to shot), a drive, and a few more, so I finally stepped back to the farthest corner of the court and let 'er rip: *Bang!*

My long jumper gave me a moment of pep, a shot glass of hope that I could pull off a comeback.

"I can't get inside. You'd think I'd be able to get inside. You'd think I'd be able to gluteus maximus my way in there," I said, frustrated, but still fully aware that I had just used a noun as a verb.

So I returned to the back of the court. Oz dared me:

"That's your shot."

Net.

Now I trailed only 5–3.

Oz countered with his signature shot. "If I hit those, we're in trouble." (I silently admired the fact that, in order to trash-talk, he choose to use "we" instead of "your sorry butt.")

I finally made a difficult inside shot with my left hand ("Nice shot, Ted!") and a couple more long ones to pull to within one, 7–6. And it was at that moment, I suspect, that Oz decided he had had enough. He scored four straight baskets, performed a gentle fist pump when he won, then hugged me and congratulated me for my mini-comeback.

"As soon as I knew your ass was so damn big and so strong, I fouled you every point and you never called it, which is why you're a gentleman," he said.

He said that the key was that he knew he had to take away my inside game, which he did with those ambidextrous, surgical hands, to force me somewhere else on the court. Offensively, he went to his strengths, and I couldn't defend. But it didn't matter— we sweated, we jawed, we competed, we had fun.

For Oz, basketball—all sports, really—is a good metaphor for everything we do, especially as we grow older.

"I think the first half of life is about learning the rules of life. So it's learning the rules of the game—the skill set you need to play the game. You play the game a little bit, but you're concerned about the rules a lot. This is metaphorically true for our lives independent of basketball," he said. "The second half of life has to be only about playing the game. It doesn't matter about rules anymore. It's about the joy that you have, where you experience that moment of connection, which we all seek as human beings. If you can do that, it's absolute bliss."

What Oz hit on so majestically in our quick game was how powerful competition could be as a form of motivation. There's no doubt in my mind that if I lived near Oz and had semiregular games with him, I would turn his butt-beating of me into a motivator. I'd train to keep up with him, I'd work on my shots, I'd get better, and I'd get smaller. He instinctually served as the perfect opponent for me.

He stepped on my throat to win the game, but somehow never made me feel that he was doing so.

The Ingredients for Lasting Motivation

Several years earlier, in an attempt to lose weight, I registered for the Disney Marathon. I followed a plan for three weeks and then bailed. I signed up sixteen, maybe twenty weeks before the race, thinking that the act of forking over triple-digit bucks would be enough to get me moving. I ran three or four times a week, but even two miles felt like twenty, so I knew there would be no way, in the time I had before race day, to prepare my body for the rigors of 26.2. Two years later, I registered for Disney again and trained for exactly three fewer weeks than I had the first time. Two big, fat fails.

It doesn't take a psych scholar to know what happened. In both cases, I was frustrated with my body, I looked for a quick fix, and I desperately hoped that the act of clicking a few buttons and entering a credit card number would jump-start some pesky brain chemicals to push my XXL frame to the starting line. Of the 532 possible ways I had either tried or thought about trying, I attempted to convince myself that this would be how I'd lose the weight.

In 2010, I did it again. This time, though, I acted like a man desperate to win a court appeal. I sent an e-mail to an editor friend at *Runner's World* and pitched him an idea for a blog called *The Marathon Virgin*, about the experiences of a first-timer trying to train for and run the long race. Considering that some half a million people finish marathons every year, I figured I could make some kind of connection with other back-of-the-packers. My main thought was that maybe *this* would be the thing that would get me moving. My editor friend quickly wrote me back and told me that the magazine got pitches like that all the time, but, sure, let's give it a try. I don't think my friend knew my ambulance-tail story from back in the day, but he certainly knew I was not a pro-totypical runner. And by "not prototypical," I mean that I looked as much like a distance runner as a Kenyan marathoner looks like a lineman. When I started *The Marathon Virgin*, I found an audi-ence that was smart, passionate, and compassionate. They wanted me to succeed. Now I had no choice.

I couldn't bail. I couldn't fail.

So what was the difference between those three years? What motivated me to try something new—to feel like I *had* to do it? Some would argue that the equation is easy: public accountability + the fear of failure + support from fellow runners = motivation. It's not as simple as that, and that's where the science and psy-chology come in: What makes us tick? What makes us want to succeed? What inspires us to move forward? And what holds us back?

Ask people why they want to get in shape, lose weight, or run a marathon, and you'll get all kinds of answers: I want to win a bet. I want to be there for my kids. I want to stop splitting seams. Flip the spotlight onto the other side of the equation, to the peo-ple like me who've never been able to turn the corner to make a sustained and permanent change, and they'll probably give you a laundry list as well: Not enough time. My knees really hurt. Have you ever actually tasted Fritos Honey BBQ Flavor Twists?

Thin line, right? The line between hitting the road and hit-ting the roadblocks?

Some research suggests that motivation, like just about every-thing else that plays a role in our gaining or losing weight, has a genetic component. One University of Missouri study, written about by Gretchen Reynolds in *The New York Times*, examined the physical behavior of rats: those that liked to run and those that didn't. Scientists separated the groups and found that there were differences in some of the genes in the areas of the brain that dealt with rewards and motivation—the implication being that some of us are hardwired to want to be active and some of us are hardwired to develop pressure sores from watching the entire series of *The Sopranos* in one shot. The study's author told *The Times* that in the future, genetic tests could conceivably ID people's inherent levels of motivation.

When it comes to brain chemistry, the main neurotransmitter involved in motivation is dopamine, which is often labeled as a feel-good chemical and plays a role in how we form habits and addictions. When we do something that feels good, dopamine is released, and in turn, we feel even better. So we get caught in this cycle: eat ice cream, feel good, want more ice cream, despite the fact that other chemical and biological reactions will make us pack on pounds. But dopamine is actually a little trickier than that.

Derek Daniels, PhD, of the University at Buffalo, told me that in recent years, dopamine has been thought of more as a "this is important" chemical, rather than just a feel-good chemical. And it's engaged when we're in states of deficits—such as hunger or thirst. "Dopamine is there to make us like food, like sex, all the things that are important for our survival as a species," Daniels said. "Those things all tap into the dopamine system." You can quench your thirst or eat when hungry. You can also stimulate hormones associated with exercise that elevate dopamine. (Note: Newer evidence suggests that endocannabinoids are the key chemicals responsible for the runner's high; drugs such as marijuana mimic the effect of endocannabinoids. This is interesting for a couple of reasons. For example, it may help explain why we have this system. "If endocannabinoids make us feel good and reduce pain, and distance running elevates these endocannabinoids, it's possible that somewhere in the history of our species, individuals who had 'good' endocannabinoid systems were able to run long distances easier, and therefore were less likely to get eaten, were more likely to be able to explore more territory looking for resources, or were more likely to survive for some other reason, making them more likely to have offspring who were also able to run long distances with less pain and more pleasure," Daniels said.)

So where does motivation come in? Essentially, you're telling your body what's important, what feels good—no matter whether it's good or bad for you healthwise. The trick, of course, is figuring out how to make the switch. How do we go from running to the fridge to running a race? How do we go from sitting to moving? How do we go from supersize to supersmall?

Experts believe that motivation comes in two forms: extrinsic and intrinsic. Extrinsic motivation can be defined as more surface-level—for example, the goal "to lose weight," or other goals tied to how others view you. Some would argue that my goal to run a marathon was more superficial than a fresh blister. At the time I made the decision, I talked to motivational expert Jay Kimiecik, PhD, a professor at Miami University in Ohio, and we discussed the various depths of motivation—the difference between, say, setting goals and being moved by something bigger.

"What are you going to do after the marathon?" he asked. "If the experience is a notch on the experience belt, what have you done with the inner work that will propel you to keep going after the experience? That's a reasonable question to ask every now and then."

His point was a good one. Was I doing this just because I wanted to write about it? Because I wanted to lose some pounds? If that were the case, motivational experts argued, I could only set myself up for failure—because those aren't intrinsic goals, that is, deeper goals driven by how you feel at an emotional, even spiritual level. Intrinsic motivators are those that you sustain over time and that serve three basic needs that we all have and that play a role in motivation. If you're fulfilling those needs, you're in a good place— being driven by intrinsic motivators. These three needs are:

- **Autonomy:** You're doing it by yourself, you're in control. Nobody's pressuring you, explicitly or otherwise, to lose weight or meet a certain goal.
- **Relatedness:** You feel a sense of community with other folks. It seems somewhat contradictory to autonomy, but it is different. Your esteem is tied to others, but you do not feel pressured or demeaned by others. You're in control but you have others for support.
- **Competence:** You find some success in whatever activity you're doing. When the scale starts moving, the miles pile up, the pants size drops, and this motivates you—because you've shown some success. The opposite is also true: When you don't see success or improvement, it's the pin to the balloon of motivation.

When I talked to the man credited with coming up with this psychological theory—it's called the self-determination theory— he told me that while we can all have different levels of the three, the secret to lasting motivation is that none of them need suffer. In fact, the first words that Edward Deci, PhD, a professor at the

University of Rochester, told me when I asked him about it were: "It's clear that all three need to be satisfied in order for [us to have] optimal performance, especially optimal well-being."

Many of us use extrinsic factors to get us going: a spouse makes a comment about weight, clothes don't fit, we make a bet with a coworker about who can drop ten pounds the fastest. These can be effective kick starts, but they're usually not enough to satisfy all three needs for the long term. The difficulty, Kimiecik said, can lie in the transition from extrinsic motivators ("I can beat you in a bet") to intrinsic ones (enjoying playing tennis because you simply love playing tennis).

"Take folks who set a goal to do a marathon. What's next? I think when that happens, they get held up on the extrinsic and don't engage in the intrinsic—the inner feeling that they get from the experience," said Kimiecik, who has himself competed in the USA Masters Track and Field Championships. "That's what propels me forward each and every day. Am I feeling I'm getting good at this? And at some point am I connecting with other people in a deeper way that this is who I am? It comes back to the intrinsic to enjoy and sustain a behavior."

Much of this, of course, is tied into goal setting—managing the balance between healthy, attainable, and challenging goals that will push you forward and those that, if not attained, will cause you to self-destruct. When I once interviewed an expert on motivation and goal setting, he told me that it also comes down to mental toughness to work around obstacles that can derail goals. When you learn and succeed, you raise your aspirations. If you fail, you have to be resilient to plow forward. Even then, setting the goal isn't enough, unless you have those three intrinsic factors revving.

"I would never ever tell people not to set goals, but if there's no deep engagement," Kimiecik said, "even achieving that goal can be a hollow experience."

Maybe the best description of the difference between extrinsic and intrinsic factors was made to me by a researcher who studies exercise motivation. With extrinsic factors, we do something (say, exercise or diet) as a means to an end. The end is the reward (or a punishment to avoid, he said). So we do things to avoid the negative feelings such as guilt or shame. With intrinsic factors, the behavior itself provides the rewards: the euphoria of exercise in and of itself motivates you to do it again. Not because of some figure on a scale or a certain dress size or time goal, but because you love the sweat, or the endorphins, or whatever goodness you feel from challenging your body.

When I told Deci, the originator of self-determination theory, about my marathon-sign-up screw-ups a few years back, he thought that in the first two cases, I was acting out because I thought that running a marathon was something I *should* do, maybe because I wanted to impress others or because I was putting some kind of pressure on myself. "My guess," he said, "is that something over the course of time changed for you so that your attitude changed about it, that this is something I want to do for myself, rather than something I should do for myself. With that change in your orientation, it's easier to keep at it."

How to Manufacture Motivation

The hard part for me has always been knowing there's no button to press to automatically choose intrinsic motivators. You can't will yourself to be motivated, I always believed. You can't tell yourself what to feel. What you hope for is to parlay those extrinsic motivators into a deeper, more meaningful purpose so that you continue to choose bananas over banana pudding, not just until January 4 or 5. What I've learned is that the opposite is more likely true. We can cook up our own motivation from scratch, and we don't have to think of it as a dichotomy, with extrinsic being bad and intrinsic good. "You can have goals that are first externally driven," said Daniel Gould, PhD, a Michigan State University professor who studies sports psychology. "But if you do well, feel good, get healthier, you feel better and it's self-fulfilling. If an obese person doesn't want to get off the couch, and some extrinsic things will get them off the couch, and then the benefits keep coming, ultimately you're shifting from extrinsic to intrinsic."

What we've learned about how some successful athletes stay motivated can translate to the weight-loss set. Setting routines helps reinforce behavior patterns and encourage steady progress toward goals to make actions feel automatic. Tim Rees, PhD, a senior lecturer at the University of Exeter who studies the social psychology of performance, told me that there seem to be four keys to staying motivated to perform well:

- **Goal setting:** It's about not just setting goals, but also developing those contingency plans I talked about in chapter 3. What if things don't go your way? What if you hit an obstacle you don't know how to get around? What if you turn your ankle ten weeks before your big race? What if just one Dorito turns into just one bag of Doritos?

- **Imagery:** Rees said that taking your articulated goal one step further—actually visualizing yourself accomplishing it—can keep motivation high.
- **Self-talk:** I know some people who think self-talk is a bunch of psychological bunk. But the reason it can work is that it helps you articulate the bigger goals in the face of derailments. I should try self-talk in the face of blueberry pie.
- **Anxiety control:** People have to realize that anxiety is normal, and that everyone experiences stresses when trying to achieve goals. "You have to try to somehow restructure how you think about stress," Rees said. For example, somebody gets bummed about a setback; that anxiety and guilt can be enough to deflate goals and put you back on the path to unhealthy eating. Instead, Rees said, the tactic should be to look back on what has been accomplished ("I've lost fifteen pounds already!"), so you can put mistakes and obstacles in context. The theory would play out like this: If three months ago I told you that you'd be fifteen pounds lighter but that you slipped up a few times along the way, you'd accept that. So don't beat yourself up for the occasional mistakes. Appreciating your accomplishments works by downgrading the importance of the stressor, so that you don't get sidetracked and can continue to work on the process of achieving your goals.

Peter Gollwitzer, PhD, the New York University goal-striving researcher, would also argue that an additional element to successful goal setting and motivation is planning. In the meta-analysis that looked at ninety-four studies involving eight thousand people, one big conclusion stuck out: Having an intention to hit a goal is not enough, and does not guarantee meeting that goal. That's because many people don't know how to deal with problems that come up during the process, but having contingency plans—the if-then mantra that he talked about—better helped participants reach their goals.

When training for my marathon in 2010, I wish I had had an if-then mantra: "If I nearly break my ankle by tripping over a ten-year-old offensive lineman during peewee football practice two months before the race, then what would I do?"

Staying on Track When You Want to Get Off

As an assistant coach on my boys' football team, I didn't know a ton about the intricacies of coaching football, but I did love helping the team, guiding them through drills, giving them the "let's go" yells from the sidelines. One summer night, I was putting the kids through a drill, sweating like a glass of lemonade on a 100-degree porch. I stepped back, got my foot caught under a fallen kid, rolled my ankle, and toppled over. I came up limping, and one of my sons said, "What about your marathon?"

I knew the ankle was bad, but with a cinched-up cleat that would stabilize it, I was able to muster through the rest of practice. Afterward, we stopped at Five Guys for a burger (surprise, surprise), and that's when I made the mistake. I slipped off my cleat, and my ankle swelled like a watermelon. I hunched over and felt sick—so sick that I didn't even order a burger (so you *know* it was bad). I could hardly walk, and I iced the ankle as soon as I got home. It was already purple; I had to see a doctor.

The X-ray showed nothing was broken, but the doc said I shouldn't run for a few weeks, though she didn't rule out my running the marathon, which was a little more than two months away. As I walked out, I felt a little desperate: I had scored a spot in the hard-to-get-into lottery of the New York City race, and I had this blog in which I had announced I would be running. In other circumstances, knowing that I'd lose three weeks of training, I probably would have deferred my participation in the race and tried for a spring marathon. But I wanted to accomplish what I had already failed at twice before—completing the training and running a marathon. I didn't want my injured ankle to be another excuse.

When I returned to running, I started slowly and then very quickly had to ramp up the miles. I was already slow and sloppy as a runner, and my injury only made things worse. I had to sacrifice some long runs, but did manage to get in one twenty-miler before race day just as my plan had called for. I had two strikes against me—my (ample) size and my (lack of) speed. But now I felt as if I had a third: my lost training and suspect ankle. By the time race day got close, I decided that I wasn't going to back out.

I stood at the start of the race that November morning and had two thoughts: How am I going to do this? Where's the closest place to the finish line that serves mashed potatoes?

As I ran (and plodded and walked that day), I appreciated all the sights, sounds, and mass of humanity out there: people either going after their goals or supporting those doing so. I saw my wife twice on the course and started tearing up when I saw her in the last stretch of the race. "Finish strong!" she cheered. "Finish strong!"

Turned out I had a long day out there. I finished, but I finished much slower than I wanted, and at a pace that, I knew, looked horrible to the outside world of runners. (It took me more than six hours.) I wanted to be happy that I'd finished, but I felt more disappointed—and embarrassed. I wanted to feel like I'd scrapped my way through after coming back from an ankle injury that should have sidelined me. I wanted to feel good. But I felt just okay. While I changed as a person after that race, one thing didn't change: my weight. I still hovered around 235 pounds. In the time leading up to the race, I had stated that my goal was to complete a marathon because I never had. It's true that it was an amazing experience—the crowds, the challenge, being passed by a juggler. I was disappointed with my time, but privately, what disappointed me most was that I'd thought that the process of training for this goal would be exactly what I needed to reach my *ultimate* goal and change my body. And that didn't happen.

I think I know what was going on deep inside my brain.

For many years, I was a part of weekly conference calls with the members of the team that produced the YOU: The Owner's Manual series of books. There were lots of folks on the team, lots of folks on the call—a collection of some brilliant thinkers, some in medicine and some not. For many of the books in the series, we talked about the Goldilocks theory of health: For optimum well-being, don't want too much or too little of anything. Find your way to the middle area and you'll live a healthy life. It's a theory that big thinker and coauthor Craig Wynett used a lot in our discussions, and he's exactly right. It applies to almost all areas of health: With food, you can't eat too much or you'll get fat, and if you get too little, your body will go into starvation mode and store fat. With sunlight, if you get too much, you'll damage your skin, but if you don't get enough, you can become deficient in vitamin D and increase your risk of cancer. With stress, if you have too much, you're at risk for many health problems, but you also need some amount of stress because it helps you face challenges and meet deadlines.

It's a classic bell curve: Stay away from the ends, put yourself in the middle, and you'll live a long and happy life without your innards dropping over your waistline.

What does that have to do with the fact that I shuffled along the streets of New York at the pace of a flat-tired tricycle? If I can Freud-up for a second, here's what I think happened in my mind: For some people (looking at myself here), there's glory at either end of the bell curve.

You win the race, or come close, and people admire you in a different way. *Whoa, he's fast. Man, she was smoking down the last 400 meters. Wow.*

You come in last or darn close, and people talk about you because they admire you. *Whoa, did you see the hips on that guy? Good for him for tackling this challenge and doing something this hard. Way to stick with it. You did it! Wow.*

I don't think I've cared much about the attention, and I know I didn't run slow on purpose, but I also believe that many of us are searching for approval when we do things that nobody thinks we can do. It's probably the reason I decided to run that first half marathon some ten years before. That was the motivation: to try something beyond my expectations.

It's probably the reason, in 2013, I signed up to do an

Ironman—a dream goal, perhaps not a realistic one. I want to take on things I'm not sure I can do. Does it increase the pressure? Does it increase the anxiety to perform? Does writing about it mean you have more at stake if you fail? Sure. But I also think those challenges serve as powerful motivators.

I've always been puzzled about the why. Why do I run? Why do I take on events I probably have no business competing in? Why do tacos always win? I think that's at the heart of all our issues—the motivation part. Deep down, we do want to change. But how do we do it? How do we translate an abstract motivating thought ("I wish I were smaller") into tangible actions day after day, over one obstacle after another?

I sign up for races because I think they will be the motivation for me finally to get in shape—that the pure act of announcing to the world that I'm going to compete will force me to make better choices. But for me, and lots of folks, that's not enough.

The drive to change, it turns out, is much more complex. Part of the weight-loss process isn't about the calorie-in, calorie-out equation, but the nuances of the brain that allow you to sustain that change. Sure, it's easy to say in a few words what motivates you: "Bikini season!" But what's not so easy is to *feel* that motivation, to turn emotion into actions and actions into that bikini, week after week. (I use *bikini* here as a universal symbol of desirous bodies, not because I know what it feels like to wear one.)

I've learned my lesson about motivation: I *thought* that motivation was the key to losing weight. With a built-in goal and public accountability, I assumed that if I did the work, the result would be a marathon finish that came with the rewards of a medal and a lighter weight. But maybe here's what happened: I tried to game the system. I tried to force motivation on myself that was a little bit beyond my reach. I created an environment in which I had no choice but to be motivated. I used that motivation to power me through the race—and I did get incredible rewards in the form of the support I felt from family, friends, and anonymous blog commenters. I also felt the satisfaction of achieving a goal that I had failed at before and, frankly, that I was unsure I could accomplish.

What that experience taught me was that, yes, you can drum up motivation to get you going. But over the long haul, that motivation has to be well grounded and deep. You can't go after one goal in the hope of achieving another. It shouldn't be "If I run the race, I'll lose weight," but rather, "If I sign up for the race, I'll do the necessary training, I'll finish the race, and if by chance I also lose weight, then that's a bonus." You have to examine why you're doing something, and what you want to get out of it, and you have to ask yourself, "Is it ever enough? What happens when I reach the goal?"

After the race, part of me felt like a failure—because of my slow time and because my shape hadn't changed all that much. I was a changed person, but not in the way I thought. What the marathon really taught me wasn't about motivation. It was about focus, it was about flexibility, and it was about this:

The goal isn't the goal. The journey is the goal.

The experience, the process, the interactions you have with people as you prepare, the card you get from your wife telling you that she believes in you, the tape job on your ankle and your wondering whether you can bounce back, the long solo training runs that start at 5:00 a.m., when you take one step and ask yourself if you have the legs to go twenty miles that day—the finish line is only the exclamation point; the real content is what happens in the sentence that leads up to it.

A few months after the race, I started a new blog for *Runner's World* called *The Big Guy Blog*, with the subtitle "An Extra-Large Runner Writes about Life in a Medium World." (I tried telling the editors they may need to add an extra *extra*.) That would pose a new set of problems. Part of my work identity was about representing the larger set. So I had to wrestle with the idea that maybe this was just who I was destined to be. I would use my weight as my blogging antagonist, and maybe that would reinforce my identity. Extra-large was just who I was—and who I would always be.

In my opening post for *The Big Guy Blog*, I decided not to commit to any more marathons for the time being, any more races, and try to focus on the process and the journey. I ended the first post this way:

> I guess I'm just trying to avoid the mistakes I've made, learn from them, and grow as a runner. I'm trying to think about several small goals, rather than one big one. Well, that's not entirely true, since I guess I do have one biggie—to get fired from this gig on the grounds that the name no longer applies.

The Smart Strategy: Make It a Game

The subject line: "Howdy." The first line: "So here's an email I've been meaning to write for a while, friend Spiker."

The e-mail came from one of my former students, a talented

writer named Joe Alewine, who served the role of—and I mean this as a compliment, because he always entertained and never disrespected—class comedian. After Joe graduated, I ran into him a few times while he worked at the local Home Depot, and we occasionally met up to talk life and careers and sports. Soon Joe up and left his job to pursue his writing goals, and I didn't keep up that much with his life until he sent that e-mail. He wrote: "I've taken up screenwriting, which I'm passionate about. I've gotten fairly good at tennis, pretty much quit drinking, become a half decent cook, and have lost nearly sixty pounds all within the last year and a half, all without ever looking at a diet book."

Even though I never considered Joe heavy, my impression of him was that he never cared much about weight—that he was as comfortable about himself as anyone, that he enjoyed beers and burgers, that it just didn't matter much if he wore a few extra pounds. He was smart, savvy, funny—and he was mature enough to place value on those things. So I wanted to know his story: the why and the how.

"I have many, many bad qualities," Joe told me when we reconnected, "but I'm not tremendously vain. I never really related to the vanity part. I just figured my grandparents were heavy and that's the way it was." Joe reached 100 pounds when he was ten, 200 when he was fifteen, and figured that the next logical step was 300 when he turned seventeen. He never got that high, but he played football and just didn't much care about how much he weighed or how he looked. His standard was one that many men share: "I just want to be able to take my shirt off and not be embarrassed." Joe told me the story of a friend, not a huge guy, who took his shirt off on the beach. A woman approached him and asked him if he worked out. When the friend said no, the woman said, "I can tell." Joe's assessment: "That doesn't really have to happen to you for you to think that it *could* happen to you."

That dialogue served as a solid example of a different kind of standard: It's not about being perfect; it's about being not embarrassed—which seems both underachieving and realistic at the same time. Using the metrics of just being able to feel decent about your body and your self-esteem, it seems, can be a lot healthier than always trying to chase perfection. Not wanting to be embarrassed can mean a whole spectrum of things, such as (a) not too fat, (b) about average, (c) "Hey, you're not half bad," and (d) "Damn, you look good." It's clearly not one of our idealized goals in the media ("Become Marginally Attractive in Six Short Days!"), but no doubt, it's an approach that has some value.

After college, Joe's weight fluctuated (when he worked at Home Depot, for example, he walked all day and ate only one meal a day and lots of beer, but the constant motion kept his weight manageable). Soon after, though, he moved back home to south Florida and grew to 260 pounds (he's six foot one). He started playing tennis with his younger and thinner brother three or four days a week and dropped ten or fifteen pounds doing that. Still, being a 243-pound tennis player meant that his brother was beating him four out of every five times they played. It reached the point where Joe's only goal was to beat his brother twice in a row, which seemed like a meek goal for an older brother.

Joe remembers the exact moment when he knew he was going to change his body. Trying to hold serve against his brother, he was down a point. On the next serve, the play ran long—he moved from corner to corner, making every shot, and finally winning the point. "But I was so gassed that I immediately lost the last two points and the game," he said. "I knew the reason was that it took so much effort to move that I was exhausted, and I knew I had to address the weight. I tried everything before—changing strings, watching YouTube videos on strategy, watching more tennis on TV. Eventually you realize it comes down to the fact that you can't get to the ball, and no strategy is going to help you get to that ball."

Joe then made changes to his diet. His adjustments included ritualizing his breakfast, weighing himself every day, snacking on a high-fiber protein bar, giving up soda, eating more spicy foods (to add flavor without adding sugar or other bad ingredients), and not using food as a reward. Before, if he won a tennis set, he'd hit the Wendy's drive-thru for a double-bacon burger and a soda. "Stopping that process was huge," he said. Instead of making his favorite foods a regular part of his diet, he ate them only every so often, which made him enjoy them even more without the guilt that came from eating them every day. "I discovered that bread and butter with chocolate milk was the greatest food—greater than the greatest steak." He also gave up his habit of watching movies with a bucket of buttered popcorn and Mexican soda.

What I love about Joe is that the food changes were only the means to what he wanted, which was to beat the crap out of his brother on the tennis court. It wasn't about the details of making it happen; it was the *reason* he wanted to make it happen. Joe has always been competitive (and that trait is only heightened against younger brothers).

"If you win at something, you feel good about yourself, and you know that the people you're dealing with (friends or kids in the neighborhood) have to treat you with respect. Wanting to compete is about wanting respect," he said. So that became the foundation for the choices he made—the ultimate goal in the strategy that psychologist Peter Gollwitzer outlined. Joe and his brother are best friends, but their competitive fire, Joe said, is what drove him. One time, when Larry was winning a lot, he made a comment to Joe: "You have an aversion to good tennis strategy."

It wasn't typical "you suck" trash talk, but rather an unintentionally condescending comment—condescending not because Larry was offering to help, but because he meant Joe *needed to be helped*.

"It got me so pissed off that I couldn't think of anything but winning," he said. "I would've chewed through an oak tree to win. I was tired of getting my ass kicked, like it was a foregone conclusion. I didn't even realize after a while that I didn't expect to win. That pissed me off more than anything."

Joe now weighs 202 pounds and beats his brother four out of every five times.

"For people who keep struggling with Diet Plan Z or that System Y," Joe said, "you have to make losing weight not about losing weight for its own sake, but about competing at something— be it tennis or basketball or cross-country or whatever's your fancy—where your weight is a factor in your success. If you find the right thing for you, your competitive fire will be the engine of discipline."

As you can tell from my performance—be it in a race or in a hoops game against Dr. Oz—I've never considered myself super-competitive when it comes to sports. I don't have to win. But I do love playing. And I do love the notion of working together as a team to try to beat other folks doing the same. When I hear somebody say, "I hate to lose," I get it, I understand that desire, but I don't get the people whose nights will be ruined if they lose a game of party Ping-Pong. I understand that the competitive fire is one of the common characteristics of elite athletes—and one of the reasons Dr. Oz so soundly whooped me on his court that day. Some love to win, and some despise to lose, but either way, that's what drives them in their training and competition. When it comes to my mild participation in recreational weekend-type sports, I've always been able to brush off a loss. Maybe that's because I never progressed very far athletically. Maybe that's because I lost 21–0 in my first racquetball game in college; she took no mercy. Maybe that's because I barely made that eighth-grade hoops team and never had my competitive fires properly stoked.

I do remember one friend saying he thought I was incredibly competitive. His statement stunned me, but Joe—a self-described wiseass who doesn't give himself enough credit for the first part of the word—crystallized it perfectly: You're competitive at things you have a shot at winning, but downgrade them as unimportant when you have none. This explains why I feel fiery when it comes to smartphone Scrabble or old-man basketball with my buddies. I can hang in there just enough to make it a game, but when it comes to anything more athletic (say, a road race), I know I'll lag so far behind that competition doesn't matter.

One time, I asked my Twitter followers if they drew more inspiration from support or snubs. Did the boos or cheers have the most impact? For sure, I thought, support would get the most support. Why wouldn't you want people slapping you on the back with "good job" cheer? Turns out, from a small sample of people who responded, that it is the jeering, the people doubting you, the tension that comes from competition, that serves as the biggest igniter. The message: *You don't think I can do it, then back the bleep off, I'll show you I can.* After all, if your supporters are cheering you on, they're probably kind enough to support you if you fail. Your doubters will only gloat when you do. The kick in the butt is more powerful than the pat on it.

It's the same message we see in some research: Competition can improve performance. Tim Rees, who studies the social psychology of performance, explained that much of the research about performance has established the importance of support systems—that, essentially, we don't live in a bubble, and that performance is affected by people around us. These studies tend to look at athletic performance, but for our purposes, there is a parallel between athletics and weight loss—in that the one trying to lose weight is engaging in a sort of public performance with his or her body. No, it's usually not done under a spotlight or in a stadium, unless you're on *The Biggest Loser*, but as we engage with family, coworkers, and friends, there is an element of public performance when it comes to weight-loss goals. Some of the more recent work, Rees explained, focuses on the role of positive and negative feedback—and how these influence performance.

What researchers have found is this: How you use positive or negative feedback (boos or cheers, trash-talking or encouragement, support or criticism) depends on who's sending the message. If positive feedback comes from someone within your inner circle, you use that to your advantage; if you receive negative feedback from someone close to you, it is more likely to derail you. But if you get negative feedback from an outsider, it can lead to better performance. In one of the studies Rees led, published in the *Journal of Experimental Social Psychology*, researchers found that criticism from foes can boost performance. In the study, participants, who were described as high-performing university athletes, threw darts blindfolded. They were then given feedback from an experimenter who was wearing a sweatshirt either from the university of those throwing the darts or from a rival university. When criticism came from rivals, subsequent performance improved (in conjunction with getting positive feedback from the insider).

"If something negative comes from somebody they don't trust, people will actively try to resist the message and show them that they're wrong," Rees said. The danger elevates when negative feedback comes from people you care about. "People who have training and exercise goals, if they're getting the message from people close to them that they'll never amount to much, they'll never be able to achieve it, people will take that and trust it and think that they must be right. But if the same message comes from outsiders—you'll never achieve that—then the response is that I'm going to prove you wrong."

The psychology makes a lot of sense when it comes to weight loss. One recent study in the journal *Obesity* found that overweight and obese teens who participated in competitive games throughout a twenty-week program lost weight, while those not involved in a competitive game didn't lose any—and actually gained weight. Participants in the study used the Nintendo Wii active video game for thirty to sixty minutes during lunch every school day, playing with one peer during the period. The activities included strength games, cardiovascular games, and sports such as basketball and tennis.

It's really the same kind of system that we see in high-profile weight-loss situations, such as on *The Biggest Loser*, a show that, while criticized for some of its methods, does use competition to help fuel motivation. The competition comes in the form of weekly tasks, but also in the big picture: financial incentive for the winner, a tactic that certainly some people have used as a way to kick-start a plan (i.e., an office bet for who can lose the most weight). This can work, because of not only the übergoal of getting healthier, but also the tangible reward that's the product of the competition. In one Mayo Clinic study, for example, people who were offered financial incentives for sticking to a weight-loss plan (and meeting a monthly weight-loss goal) lost an average of about nine pounds compared to those who were offered no incentives (these lost an average of a little more than two pounds).

This method can work whether or not you're doing it with people close to you. If you do it with people close to you, you have the support and encouragement, and friendly rivalries within the group, so you're motivated to do well. Do the same competition with a group of coworkers or maybe even strangers (through such things as community contests), and your drive is dictated not just by motivation to do well, but also by a desire to show the others that you can win, that you are the alpha. The danger comes, the research would suggest, if the group you think supports you turns on you. And that can be the trickiest part of using competition or anger or testosterone to power weight-loss efforts.

Take the case of the drill instructor trainer, someone who yells, screams, pushes, makes you feel like a pile of steaming cow dung if you can't do twelve push-ups—in essence, that person creates a competitive environment, sparking in you an "I'm gonna show him" attitude. "That may work for some and be devastating for others," said researcher Daniel Gould.

Gould's point—that we all respond to competition differently—reminded me that competition can be interpreted in a lot of different ways. Competition can be defined in the traditional way (me versus you in some game, contest, or challenge). It can also be defined as a little softer (competing in a new-to-you challenge with friends for charity). Competition can be internal (asking yourself if you can win the day, win the meal, hit a goal, beat your goal). In life, we tend to see people who fall into the extreme cases— people who have to win absolutely everything they do, and people who couldn't care less about winning or losing or even engaging in any kind of type of me-versus-you scenario. The reality, Gould said, is that in terms of how we use competition to spur us on, most of us fall somewhere inside that spectrum.

The reason that integrating some form of competition into a weight-loss strategy can work is because of exactly what my friend Joe said: It takes the diet away from the diet itself—there's a higher-order goal in play. That holds true whether you're a man or a woman, whether you're inherently competitive or not. We can all find ways to have some kind of competition—from traditional duels (such as sports) to quieter and more introspective competition (such as beating your daily pedometer reading).

You want your body to function better. You want to perform better. You want to do, to live, to engage. And if you can find some way to do it—weekly basketball games, tennis matches, a weight-loss bet, signing up for a race that's beyond your perceived abilities in order to have an inner competition with yourself—it can work on two levels: not only by making you focus on the competition rather than a diet, but also because of the power and energy you can draw from involving other people in your quest, as friend, foe, or both.

Truth: You Can Dream
Your Own Diet

I had worked at *Men's Health* for only about a year when the editorial team held an off-site retreat to brainstorm ideas and talk about the future of the magazine. Early on during my time there, I stayed under the radar, did my job, didn't make waves, just tried to plow ahead, learn the ropes of health writing, and hope to live up to the expectations of some of the most creative and smart people I'd ever worked with.

Most of the *Men's Health* team were also fit and lean—regular marathoners, lifters, ball players, and overall excellent athletes, no matter their age. The two guys I worked most closely with, however, were a little less like the others and a little more like me. One, although thin, didn't like exercise, and didn't eat vegetables. Another enjoyed his food and beverages as much as I did, and also used his chubbier-than-the-rest-of-the-office body as the butt of his own jokes. Me? I was the biggest of the bunch, and during our lunchtime jaunts, I had quickly established a reputation as someone who could suck up a plate of food with the velocity of an industrial-size car vac.

During the retreat dinner, one of our smartest writers, Greg, commandeered the conversation to establish the fact that nobody anywhere (ever, in the history of all the land!) could eat faster than he could. Now a TV personality and one of the funniest folks I've worked with, Greg would walk up and down the office halls and joke in a louder-than-conversational voice, "Spiker! Why aren't you wearing any pants?" I always wore pants.

All muscle and quite possibly half my weight, Greg could indeed put it away. But when he declared at that dinner that he was the Indy 500 of eaters, I saw the corners of my friends' mouths move upward ever so slightly. They grunted an indignant laugh, as if to say, "Son, keep talking." One of them mentioned my name, suggesting that if Greg wanted to put his money where his mouth was, they knew a guy, and he happened to be sitting right here next to them. I felt like a boxer, not saying a word, just letting my handlers promote a matchup. Two heavyweight appetites going gut-to-gut. As Greg kept talking, the room started buzzing. Now the whole staff wanted to see this happen. They wanted to see if the under-the-radar underdog could dethrone the beating-his-chest champion.

Greg continued with Ali-like verbiage. Nobody—*noooobody*—faster.

Dinner had finished while the peak of jabbering took place, so it was decided that the battle would have to take place over whatever the host restaurant was going to bring out for dessert.

Guys being guys, the rest of the team—maybe fifteen or twenty editors and writers, most of whom were men—arranged for Greg and me to sit face-to-face for this Thrilla of Vanilla. The server brought us each a plate dotted with four fist-size desserts. This wasn't about quantity. This was purely about speed.

I can't tell you a thing about any of the four items, what they looked like or tasted like—I think they resembled mini-éclairs (puff pastry, some cream, surely some chocolate icing)—but I can tell you this:

Just a few seconds after the "Go!" sounded, I had finished.

No chewing, no tasting, no mercy. KO, in the first round.

As Greg looked up, stunned, I looked him in the eye, raised my plate, then licked it dry in a final, taunting display of never-seen-before bravado.

The room erupted.

He had the bigger mouth, but I had the faster one.

Greg knew he'd lost, and there was no denying whose tongue had just Cascaded the plate.

That's sort of what my relationship with food has been like: Food is part of who I am. I eat fast. I eat a lot. And that, I presume, has been part of my persona projected to the outside world—not being embarrassed about enjoying my meals.

I have nobody to blame for the way my food has set up camp on my body. I know I eat too much. I know I eat too quickly. I know I often make choices that aren't best for my body. But I spent much of my life doing it. Because I like tacos. And I like ice cream. And I find myself living with the consequences of the way I eat and trying to make adjustments so I can have a better body. I want to have my cake and eat yours, too.

While I have had these moments that are beyond the reasonable approach to eating, it's typically not how I live most of my life. I don't usually gorge on chips, I try to not order the side of fries (in fact, I rarely order fried foods), and I do always keep a watchful eye over portion sizes (a battle I often lose). This is the dilemma many of us have: Deep down, we know what we should be eating. We know that grilled is better than fried, chicken is better than candy, and vegetables are better than puffy-air snacks that have orange finger residue with the eye-searing tint of hazardous waste. But there's so much more that goes into eating well, eating right, eating better. Perhaps Jonathan Bailor, author of *The Calorie Myth*, said it best: "It's simple, but it's not easy."

Changing Our Eating Is About Changing Our Environment

I know I may be an exception when it comes to food-consumption pedigree: Not everybody who battles with weight issues is a shovel-it-in-as-fast-as-you-can eater. Some people are sugar addicts. Some people eat because they're bored or because it's fun to binge-eat while you binge-watch *Homeland*. Some people eat well most of the time, but lose control when their lives do the same. Part of figuring out how to eat better comes down to identifying your triggers, your weaknesses, and the reasons you eat—beyond the obvious ("Uh, cinnamon buns good"). That's largely what the first part of this book is about: figuring out the more complex issues involved in our eating. After that, it's a bit easier to handle the nutrition part of it—I say "a bit" easier because, in our current environment, it's *really* hard to avoid crap.

In 2012, Peter Attia, MD, cofounded the Nutrition Science Institute (NuSI) with science journalist Gary Taubes with the goal of reducing the individual, social, and economic costs associated with obesity-related diseases. In school, Attia studied engineering, but switched paths to become a doctor. He entered medical school thinking he was going to become a pediatric oncologist, but soon found that surgery was his passion. In his personal life, Attia excelled as an athlete, having been a boxer, and as an adult, he swam the Catalina Channel in both directions (from Catalina Island to Los Angeles, and, on a separate occasion, the way back). Even when he was exercising for three or four hours a day, his weight rose—up to 205 pounds with 25 percent body fat. He thought he was doing it right (exercising, staying away from fast food), but he carried fifty pounds of fat, and his blood numbers suggested that he had metabolic syndrome (a collection of signs, including cholesterol and blood sugar, that suggest insulin resistance). Soon, he radically changed his diet: He eliminated most sugar, and he swapped out white carbohydrates for brown ones. Later, he reduced his starches to one serving per day (though fruits and vegetables were unlimited); he reduced his carb intake dramatically, had an average required protein intake, and had a high fat intake. When he started this change, he was at 195 pounds, and two years later he was down to 170 pounds and 7.5 percent body fat. Attia said making the changes wasn't difficult physiologically, but was logistically tough during the first few months because sugar (in all its forms) is so ubiquitous. Reading labels and substituting things, like real pasta sauce for the jarred, store-bought kinds, took time.

When I spoke with Attia, I had just listened to a TED Talk he'd given—an emotional one in which he admits to silently blaming a diabetic patient for her condition, and then challenging the audience to rethink its beliefs about obesity: Maybe it isn't food that's triggering hormonal changes that are making us fat, but hormonal changes are triggering us to eat the wrong kinds of foods? What if everything we assume to be true is all wrong? One of Attia's missions with NuSI is to let science do its job and figure out the answers to some questions we only think we know the answers to. Attia's mission now is to help us all flip the switch—to understand nutrition principles, yes, but more important, to help change the nutritional environment we live in.

Attia told me the best comparison to use when thinking about the obesity situation is the history of smoking (though he admits this is an oversimplification). In the late 1940s and early 1950s, more than half the U.S. population smoked cigarettes. Research about smoking's effect was either ambiguous or unknown, Attia explained, and the tobacco industry basically said not only that smoking was not bad for you, but that it was actually good for you. That message evolved, of course (with more research indicating that smoking resulted in emphysema and lung cancer), to the point where now fewer than 20 percent of Americans smoke. The metathemes apply to food, Attia said. First, the information about smoking became clear and unambiguous, and second, the message was reinforced repeatedly. The third theme is perhaps the most important when it comes to food: "What people don't appreciate is that the environment changed so that the default no longer was to smoke," Attia said.

The environment changed from one in which we'd send cigarettes to our soldiers as rewards to one in which (a) smoking was banned in the workplace, (b) it was banned from most public places, and (c) cigarettes became heavily taxed. So now the default state is not to smoke. That doesn't mean you can't smoke. That doesn't mean that your freedoms are taken away. It means that it's harder to smoke than it is not to smoke. Attia said, "These forces matter." When it comes to food, he added, we're in a similar toxic environment that resembles one in the earlier days of smoking.

"I don't think the information we have is necessarily correct and it's not validated scientifically, but it's also potentially incorrect. We live in an environment where the default is probably driving you to eat the wrong things," he said. His examples: A two-liter bottle of water is more expensive than a two-liter bottle of soda, and advertising is catered to the socioeconomically disadvantaged. Any individual can opt *out* of the bad choices, Attia said, but the ideal state would be one in which we have to opt *in* to them—that is, one in which it takes more effort to do the unhealthy thing than the healthy thing.

"You want to make the best behaviors the default," Attia said. "We all believe in having our freedoms, and you can do what's bad for you as long as you're not hurting someone else. But perhaps you have to make an extra effort, like you have to step outside if you want to smoke. We do not need a nanny state, but it should be the case that getting a salad is the default, and maybe you have to go to the back of the store to get the chips."

One of the tough parts about the food debate is that, unlike smoking, we need food. So while we can say "stop smoking," we can't say "stop eating"—and this creates a sort of substitution system. "When you demonize one food, you have to replace it with another. When you take out saturated fat, you put something in, and that something has been more sugar and refined carbs," Attia said. Creating a healthy environment relies on having the information on what the best and worst foods are. For a long time, dietary fat was viewed as the villain; saturated fat was demonized as the cause of obesity. That story is shifting. "The evidence is certainly mounting against sugar," Attia said, "but I don't know with any great certainty that the jury is back and the case is closed."

That's really what lies at the heart of the frustration for so many of us. We want to pinpoint the dietary reason we're fat. Part of my point, I hope, is that it's about not just the food, but all the other factors that play a role in why and how much we eat. So can we say that sugar is the problem? We can certainly say we eat too much of it, and we can say that it's a huge contributor to our collective hugeness. Can we then make the leap to say that if you just eliminate all the sugar in your diet, you will forever have the body you want? Probably not.

This is why so many people are frustrated by nutrition, said Adam Bornstein, author of many diet and health books, including *Man 2.0 Engineering the Alpha*. Adam, a former student of mine, is one of the smartest people I've met when it comes to fitness and nutrition—he used to come to class with Tupperware containers of large portions of scrambled eggs. Adam has always taken a balanced approach to nutrition, not blaming any one factor. "It's a fluid science," he said. "People are always jumping the gun on the villains—saturated fat, high fructose corn syrup, gluten. The yo-yo diet cycle is created by those who jump to conclusions so fast. It's not that the science is bad—it's that the application was overgeneralized." A main theme in much of Adam's work is that while science provides a strong backbone, we as individuals also have to do some experimentation to find what works—reducing sugar, if you eat too much of it, is one step, but only one.

The First Change: Reduce Sugar

Daniel E. Lieberman, PhD, a professor of human evolutionary biology at Harvard University, wrote in *The Story of the Human Body* that an evolutionary perspective helps explain why we have a collective weight problem; while it's a multifaceted problem, too much sugar is one of the reasons. Because excessive sugar in the bloodstream is toxic, Lieberman wrote, animals evolved to convert it into fat, so we could then use that as energy when food was scarce. "Simply put, humans evolved to crave sugar, store it and then use it," he wrote. "For millions of years, our cravings and digestive systems were exquisitely balanced because sugar was rare." In other words, cavemen didn't have Count Chocula trees.

When food sources were limited, our bodies balanced out what we were ingesting with how much we were using as fuel. It's one of the reasons a growing number of people have embraced what's called the Paleo diet (or some variation thereof), eating the way our ancestors ate. When I talked to Lieberman, he cautioned that it's not simply about reverting to caveman ways.

"You have to be careful about this logic. Just because the hunter-gatherer did this, that, or the other doesn't mean it's necessarily healthier," he said. "Because natural selection only favored features that improved reproductive success, we didn't necessarily evolve to be healthy. So what our ancestors ate and did is not necessarily a road map for what we should eat and do."

Most pudding-stained fingers still do point to sugar as being the major culprit in our diet, for a couple of reasons: First, the sheer quantity of what we consume. According to the Centers for

Disease Control and Prevention, men consume 335 calories a day of added sugar, while women consume 239 calories—both equating to about 13 percent of their diets. Added sugar would include things such as white sugar, brown sugar, corn syrup, and fructose sweeteners. Second, the chemical changes caused by one of our major sources of sugar, fructose. Fructose is metabolized differently from glucose, and because of the way it's processed in the liver, it can produce the triglycerides that are stored in our fat cells, which, when dumped into our bloodstream, create a sort of chemical havoc in the form of things such as high blood pressure and insulin resistance. This insulin factor is a crucial one: Your body produces insulin to cart off the glucose that has been converted from the food you eat. When you eat too much, your body produces too much insulin and your cells can't keep up with the load, meaning that glucose ends up wandering around your blood like a lost puppy. When that lost puppy needs to find a place to stay, it hunkers down in your body as fat. Third, because of the way we use sugar so quickly, our energy levels bounce up and down more than a trampolining toddler. We're tired, we eat, we're amped, we quickly crash, we're tired, we don't want to move, we eat more, crash again, and the cycle continues. Still, the real issue here is the quantity of sugar we eat: All foods can cause a jump in blood sugar and insulin if you eat too much of them.

It's not as if there's an easy out. It's hard to give up our sugar fix, because of sugar's addictive nature, in that it releases that feel-good hormone dopamine. In one study published in the journal *Neuroscience & Biobehavioral Reviews*, researchers showed that rats exposed to excessive sugar exhibited similar behaviors to those who had drug addictions (in that they binged within the first hours of being exposed to the sugar, and they also experienced withdrawals and cravings). Bailor said, "Clinical studies show that high doses of sugar have analogous effects as morphine, heroin, cocaine—stimulating the same area of the brain. Anyone who doesn't believe it, try to give up sugar and starch and you will go through headaches because you are addicted." For example, in one recent study published in *Current Biology*, researchers tested rats by delivering a drug to the area of the brain called the neo-stratum. When they did that, rats ate twice the number of M&Ms than normal. At the same time, chemicals that induced a desire to eat also increased. The researchers compared the effect to that which occurs when drug addicts see drugs: A visual cue triggers an impulse and has an addicting effect.

One of the best looks at the nature of our addictive food substances was a piece by Michael Moss in *The New York Times Magazine*. Moss spent four years looking at the food industry and talking to more than three hundred people; the billboard on his story was this: "It's not just a matter of poor willpower on the part of the consumer and a give-the-people-what-they-want attitude on the part of the food manufacturers. What I found . . . was a conscious effort—taking place in labs and marketing meetings and grocery-store aisles—to get people hooked on foods that are convenient and inexpensive."

To be fair, lots of things can be addictive—ranging from things with potentially harmful effects (alcohol and nicotine) to those considered healthy for us (exercise and sex). And that's why the argument about sugar may not center on the sugar per se, but rather on all the environmental factors that nudge us to consume more of it. So does that make our diet issue nutritional or behavioral? Or social? Or environmental? The takeaway is that many of us are up against a gargantuan industry that economically benefits from our constantly craving bad food. This is why Attia's umbrella principles about creating the right nutritional environment could serve as the foundation for what needs to change for us to see a sizable shift in our obesity stats. If we're swimming in polluted nutritional waters, it's damn hard to consume the clean stuff if everything around us is toxic. That will be a big boat to turn, and that's one of the reasons I admire people like Attia. To change the system will take strength, science, and a public (with strong leaders) willing to fight back. In the meantime, the question is whether we as individuals can take Attia's principles and apply them to our own lives. Can we individually create environments where the default is to eat well, where we'd have to opt in to eat poorly? It's certainly one of the tactics that weight-loss experts suggest we use: Keep only good foods in your home, plan your meals, and if you eat out, know ahead of time what you're going to order that's relatively healthy. These are all about creating environments in which the default state is to eat well.

Now, Bailor believes that we've spent too much time thinking about quantities and not enough about quality. The problem is that when you focus on quantity, you start looking not at food, but at what he calls "edible products"—that is, all the processed junk we can eat, but not real food, not anything we'd find naturally from the earth. If we can make that shift away from edible products to real food—that is, nothing that needs any manufacturing, including grains—then we won't need to do things like count calories or perform any other task designed to help us manage our caloric intake.

"If you just eat real food—things you can directly find in

nature—your body automatically balances calories," Bailor said.
"Your body will balance those calories out over the long term,
just as it balances out blood pressure, your breathing rate, your
sleep cycle." Real food means that you're not messing with your
body's desire to find homeostasis—energy balance between what
you take in and what you burn off. Real food, Bailor said, allows
your body to balance out automatically; artificial and processed
edible products do not. "There's no question that of the fifty
thousand or so edible things you can find in the grocery store,
ninety-five percent are edible products that have been manufac-
tured to pleasure us, as well as to please the profit margins of
companies that manufacture them. They're all basically the same
toxic and addictive ingredients just mushed together in thousands
of different permutations. The idea that there are even that many
things is ridiculous. How are there even new foods, when there's
no new species of plants or animals? How is it that there are a
hundred new choices every year?" (This is about the point in our
conversation when I started feeling guilty about how excited I got
when I learned there was cake-batter-flavored coffee creamer.)

While some may argue that we don't definitely know everything there is to know about obesity causes and cures, few diet
experts would argue against eating whole and natural foods. This
should be a given for long-term, healthy eating—not just weight-
wise but health-wise. After all, there are plenty of stories of people
who lost dozens of pounds eating only fast food, for example, and
those people did so most likely because they found healthier options, but also because they limited calories, which can certainly
work, especially in the short term. Given how the yo-yo nature
works, that's tough to sustain for the long haul, because those bad

foods and ingredients almost *make* you eat more eventually. To be fair: If you consume too much healthy food, you can gain weight. While this might seem to contradict the calorie-balancing argument to some degree, my point isn't that you shouldn't eat these healthy foods; it's that you can't rationalize boulder-size portions with a "but they're healthy foods" argument, which some of us have been known to do. (Sheepishly raises hand.)

Bailor uses the acronym SANE for the way he believes we should classify foods:

Satiety: foods that fill us up quickly and for a long period of time;
Aggression: how quickly what we eat turns into the substances that we either use for energy or whether those calories will get stored (unaggressive is what we want);
Nutrition: how many nutrients they contain per calorie;
Efficiency: how well our bodies metabolize foods (inefficiency is good because your body has to burn more energy metabolizing them).

These are the foods that are best using the SANE framework:

- Nonstarchy vegetables (those that you can eat raw, though you don't have to), such as lettuce, kale, spinach, mushrooms, cucumbers, zucchini, and squash.
- Nutrient-dense sources of protein, such as seafood, chicken, turkey, and some cuts of red meat.
- Whole-food and healthy fats such as avocado, flax, coconut, and eggs.
- Low-fructose fruits such as berries and citrus foods such as oranges, lemons, and limes.

"Here's what's brilliant about them," Bailor said. "We desire four flavors: sweet, salty, savory, and bitter. And every single one of those flavors can be enjoyed in mass and guilt-free from whole foods. You like fruit pies, use coconut and almond flour to make a crust and whole fruits with a natural sweetener like stevia. Enjoy that and not feel guilty about it."

His remark "and not feel guilty about it" strikes me as a key phrase in this battle, for those of us addicted to sugar or who snack too much or who can eat seventy-six ounces of meat at one time. Can you find the spot where it's okay to dabble in bad foods if you eat enough of the good? Is it okay to cheat just once in a while?

"If the question is 'Can you smoke once a week, is there anything wrong with that?' I think the answer is probably not," Attia told me. "But I think the question is, can you be content smoking one cigarette a week and is that all you need to scratch the itch? Can you stop there? It's a personal decision."

Attia works with people all the time, some who can go cold turkey and give up any food—basically having the same attitude as an alcoholic who knows he can't have one drink because it'll lead to infinite drinks—and others who have the discipline to work in one bad meal a week and leave it at that. The problem is that most of us aren't able (or don't choose) to live with that kind of moderation mind-set.

"I always caution people that one bad meal a week can lead to two bad meals a week and that can lead to one bad day a week and then two days a week," Attia said. "And that's how recidivism works. I look forward to the day when you can have all the cake and ice cream on your birthday (but just not day in and day out), so that it predisposes you to health and not illness."

Bailor thinks that you can take an even broader step back when it comes to these so-called cheat meals or cheat days—that, ideally, if you eat the right foods in the right balance, to satisfy those four taste urges, you shouldn't even feel tempted to stray.

"In relationships, when you meet the right person, you don't say, 'Oh, it's so hard not to cheat on that person,'" he said. "And when you find the right relationship with food, you feel no need to cheat. This is what you were meant to do; cheating implies what you're doing is not sustainable and not fulfilling."

This concept of cheating is how some American diet programs have worked: If we assume that we know the basics of proper eating—and most of us would agree that the four SANE food groups make sense, the only hot-button issue being what role carbohydrates can play in a diet—then the formula is about constructing a plan that allows you the best chance to eat those foods. While certainly some diets are built on a foundation of "eat this and this only" (think of the protein- and fat-based Atkins diet), many other popular plans and programs are not about the food as much as about giving you a framework for eating the food. Weight Watchers (count your points) works for people who like to track their amounts. And while it has been shown to be a very successful method, because the better-for-you foods are naturally lower in points (and thus encourage participants to eat healthier), there's still wiggle room to allow people to save their points to indulge in sinful foods. Other diets encourage cheat meals and cheat days, likely because of the psychological reward that comes with this—"If I can just eat right for twenty meals, twenty-one will be noodle-rama." This is similar to one of the more promising eating methods that's gained popularity over the last few years: intermittent fasting. The basic concept of IF is this: You take regular and predetermined periods of fasting throughout the week. Some may fast for twenty-four hours once or twice a week, while others may eat during an eight-hour window every day, leaving a sixteen-hour period of fasting (that window includes sleep). This, some research would suggest, creates hormonal changes that maximize your ability to lose fat. In almost any of these or other methods, eating the right foods is the central character, but the supporting character—and the X factor—is the lifestyle and behavioral methods you use to maximize the chance that you'll eat the right foods and keep the wrong ones to a minimum or eliminated altogether.

Despite the fact that we know what to eat, the fact that we have so many people with weight problems and so many different possible solutions and programs may mean that it's not as much about the food as it is about all the other swirling factors—some of them psychological, some of them logistical, some of them physical, some of them environmental, and all of them frustrating.

At one point, I asked Attia what he ate on a typical day. I know the general ratios—most of what he consumes comes from protein and fat. But he didn't tell me the specifics of his meals because he doesn't like the N of 1 (which refers to a clinical trial in which there is only one patient)—that is, anecdotal evidence that somehow implies that's what everyone should be doing. He's regretted doing blog posts in which he's talked about his personal strategies; those are the ones that get the most attention, but they're also the ones that are not backed up by science. He understands the power of the anecdote, but also thinks that's the tragedy of today's weight-loss dogma: If you read a story of a person who lost weight eating nothing but potatoes and popcorn, the message is that this can work. "You're going to find an N of 1 for everything, but if we relied on an N of 1 to make a strong recommendation, we would still think that the earth was flat and the sun still rotated around it. We need to resist the temptation to cave in for the desire of the anecdote."

Create Your Own Diet

When it comes to nutrition, resisting anecdotal evidence lies at the heart of our dilemma. We need science to find out answers. But with such "fluid science," as Bornstein calls it, we don't have the answers—or we oversimplify them. Which means that essentially we're creating our own anecdotes, our own formulas, our own diets—which can fail miserably, of course, but may also be the way we come up with at least our own solutions.

So, yes, I believe that most people who need to lose weight could construct their own eating plan using the foundation principles that point to proper nutrition: They know they should eat lean meats and vegetables, and they know that gooey desserts aren't diet foods. While there are some gray areas—most notably with regard to carbs—most of us have a sense of what's best and what's not. But something that Attia told me also strikes me as important: We haven't figured out the answer. Some of that uncertainty has to do with specific foods and how they interact with the body, and some of it has to do with all those external and environmental factors that influence decision making, even when you know what is best for your body. Because of those unknowns, I believe, the person who is most successful at losing and maintaining weight creates an answer that combines not only scientific principles that work, but also personality principles: How do you best ensure that you can eat well?

In total, I've lost about eighty pounds from my highest weight. The drops didn't come all at once, and I've hit several plateaus for long periods, bumped up a bit at times, then dropped some more. The hardest pounds I had to lose were those last ones—the ones that took me from 220 to 200. And while I could stand to lose more, I'm comfortable and happy right around the double-century mark. Throughout the entire process, I didn't employ one strategy or follow one diet. I combined a number of tactics, nutritionally and behaviorally, to get there. As someone who writes and reads a lot of diet books and articles, I like the idea of combining traits from different plans. But some people prefer to be told to do *a*, *b*, and *c* to get results *x*, *y*, and *z*. And that's okay: If you're the kind of person who does better following a strict plan, then that tactic may work for you. At some point—because of unforeseen circumstances—it's easy to fall off strict plans, which then risks derailing the whole plan (at least in the mind of the person following it). So instead, we need big principles to follow. And that may mean cobbling together your own approach to eating.

Does that mean you should do exactly what I did? No, but it may give some clues into eating habits and principles that can work. The main message is: Create your own answer. If something stops working, try something else. If you're going out of your mind because you can never, ever, ever, ever, ever have a piece of chocolate, create your own system that allows you to indulge a little before you break down and gorge on a 4,000-calorie, seven-foot-high chocolate explosion served at a chain restaurant.

These are the principles and tactics I found to be the most

effective for losing weight, breaking through plateaus, and maintaining a healthy weight:

I Don't Believe "A Calorie Is a Calorie," but I Do Believe Calories Matter.

I, and many others, have had success counting calories. And I believe counting calories can be an incredibly effective tactic, because it keeps you aware of the quantity you're eating, gives you a tangible motivational system to follow, and teaches you that if you eat better foods, you can have more of them within a daily calorie total. There's no question that calories matter. If you eat a lot and can't burn them all up (be it through movement or your own genetic rate of metabolism), your body will store the excess as fat. However, tracking calories and thinking about calories are different from believing that every calorie is created equal. That's because the effect that foods have on our bodies, as Jonathan Bailor explained, is different: Highly processed carbohydrates increase blood sugar and insulin, which makes you store more fat. Some research shows that ingredients in processed foods change hormonal levels, increasing appetite. This causes a vicious cycle: eat bad, want more, eat more bad. One discussion held during an annual meeting of the American Association for the Advancement of Science featured panelists who discussed why we shouldn't treat every calorie as equal and how we've gotten the whole system wrong. According to a *Wired* report of that discussion, the reason the system's flawed, the panelists said, is because calorie numbers don't account for the whole digestive process—how much energy it takes to digest food or how the properties of foods may influence how they're absorbed. Essentially, processed foods are easy to digest (meaning they burn off less energy when they travel through) than foods such as beans, which require more energy to digest (thus decreasing the amount of energy that would be stored as fat). This is what's called the thermic effects of food— that is, for every calorie of protein we eat, about 30 percent of that is used up in the metabolic process, while carbohydrates use only about 5 percent during metabolization. Calorie counting need not be eliminated as a method for eating better foods and smaller amounts of them, but it should serve more as a guiding principle for the kinds of food to concentrate on. Calories matter, but that doesn't mean that every one of them should be treated equally.

I Emphasize Protein, Don't Fear Fat, and Have Learned to Bulk Up on the Vegetables.

If you're going to be successful, you have to find the healthy foods that you can eat, do like, and can fill up on. I subscribe to a lot of what Bailor and Attia talk about in terms of best choices: protein, such as chicken and red meats (I try to eat more fish, but I usually fail), fat, and vegetables. For many folks, the inclusion of non-starchy vegetables is the key: They add bulk to your plate, keep you full, and are low in calories. (Add some garlic and olive oil, roast them, and you're good to go.) For many people who fear fat, this can be a hard concept to wrap your head around: Fat doesn't make you fat. The reason: Fat doesn't trigger the insulin response (in which energy is stored as fat) as easily as carbohydrates do. Much of the credit for challenging traditional notions about fat in the mainstream media, and for focusing on carbs as the culprits in the weight-gain problem, goes to Gary Taubes, the science journalist who wrote *Good Calories, Bad Calories*. His 2002 article in *The New York Times*, "What If It's All Been a Big Fat Lie?" outlined the challenges to low-fat dieting, once thought of as the answer to obesity. In fact, it may have been the problem. There are many benefits to eating fat, including the satiety argument, in that fat helps keep you full. These days when I construct my plate, I try to get it as close to the SANE foods that Bailor recommends: Tip the scales *toward* protein, vegetables, and fats, and *away* from sugars and simple carbs.

I Don't Eliminate Carbs; I Just Reduce the Heck out of Them.

Some people say you need to get rid of all of the carbs, while others swear that there's nothing wrong with them. What I've found is that if I want to keep weight off or lose it, I need to reduce carbs drastically. Taubes's work is especially important for our thinking about carbs as the way we gain weight and store fat. But even if we accept the premise that we should avoid carbs, the bridge from solution to action is what's at play. Can you get rid of them? Do you even need to? After all, there are plenty of lean people who eat plenty of carbs. I know that I'll never fully get rid of carbs, so I don't pretend to (only to set myself up for failure). What I've found *for me* is that if I can limit them, my body does get smaller. So I try to limit them to special occasions or just a small portion here or there. After all, I do like an occasional pizza slice or a more-than-occasional glass of alcohol, and mashed potatoes are my Kryptonite. I don't *want* to give them up forever. I also don't have to have them all the time, and I don't have to have a carb just to have a carb. If I want pancakes, I may have just a few bites—or treat myself to a plate if I have had an especially long or hard workout. And I certainly had a lot of them while doing the long training for endurance events. Otherwise, I try to make my carbs of the whole-grain variety that have more nutrients and fiber than the simple no-nutrient variety. When I eat those, I treat them like . . . well, treats. I've learned to minimize carbs, and in the process, I've minimized myself.

So the big question, it seems, is how do you do that? How do you go from a Hoover-acting hog to limiting the breads and desserts and weekly trips to Dairy Queen? For me it all has to do with the next point.

I Found Substitutions.

The unofficial number one reason diets fail? We miss our favorite foods. Eventually we go back to them in large quantities and regular intervals. This isn't love, after all. (*If you love Fudgsicles, then set them free!*) This is temptation. And to deal with it, as we know, you have to have a plan: If you're going to eliminate something, you have to replace it with something. If I want something to pick at, such as a bag of chips, I use a bowl of chilled grapes; they're crunchy and sweet. If I want something a little less sweet, I may use a hard-boiled egg and olives stuffed with garlic and a small piece of chicken to hold me over. And if I want something sweet, which I do just about every night, I go to the creation that my friend Adam Bornstein taught me: protein ice cream. Mix Greek yogurt, a little almond butter, and protein powder. It whips up real nice, and if you put it in the fridge or freezer for a few minutes, it will thicken up to the consistency of ice cream. I add

berries, crushed pecans, and just a few chocolate chips. This satis-
fies my sweet cravings without all the added junk in just about
every other option I would otherwise choose. Still, if there's
something I *really* want, I'll have it; I'll just limit portion size.
More important, I'll save it for when I really, really want it, rather
than when I feel I deserve it or some other kind of sin food every
single day. After a few weeks, your substitutions become the new
normal.

I Like Intermittent Fasting.

A few years ago, Adam also taught me about intermittent fasting.
Essentially, it is a way of eating that, its proponents would argue,
encourages weight loss by putting your body in temporary modes
of fasting. It's a hot topic, the subject of much debate, and essentially calls into the question the popular diet mantra that we
should eat small meals throughout the day. While there are a few
ways to practice intermittent fasting, one of the more common
methods is eating all your meals within an eight-hour window
every day, which leaves you in fasting mode for sixteen hours
(some of that, granted, is in sleep, so it doesn't feel like sixteen
hours). Another popular way to do IF is with twenty-four-hour
fasts once or twice a week—that is, if you finish your last meal at
7:00 p.m. on Wednesday, your next meal doesn't come until the
same time on Thursday. I've tried this a few times but prefer the
eight-hour window of eating. I've never been a huge breakfast
eater—meaning that I typically make my eating window between
1:00 p.m. and 9:00 p.m. (though I do give myself some flexibility
there), so it didn't take a lot for me to give up that meal. While

there's still a lot of research that needs to be done to determine intermittent fasting's effectiveness, research seems to indicate that fasting for small periods such as these does not slow metabolism (longer fasts would), and the short periods could improve insulin sensitivity (a good thing) and reduce insulin levels, which could allow you to eat more carbs, burn fat, and not gain weight. It's not for everyone—my wife, for example, would get headaches if she didn't eat early in the day—but it's a method that I think is worth trying, especially if you like having a few carbs in your life.

I Drink a Lot.

To get me through the morning, I drink coffee, usually a twenty-four-ouncer. To get me through the afternoon, a typical witching hour, I drink a few smaller cups. (I use almond milk as much as I can, maybe a bit of low-fat milk or cream, and I do include a teaspoon or two of sweetener, using the natural sweetener stevia as much as possible.) I drink water the rest of the day. I'm not rigid about trying to hit sixty-four ounces of it a day, but it's what I'll have with every meal and when I don't have a cup of coffee on my desk. You're likely well aware of the benefits of drinking water. A German study review published in *The American Journal of Clinical Nutrition* found that while there were inconsistent results among people who drank a lot of water while dieting, there is some evidence that it can aid in reaching dieting goals.

Focusing on these two drinks helps me in a couple of ways: One, it takes the edge off if hunger comes, making it less likely that I'll reach for an unhealthy food. Two, it gives me something to do, something to keep my mouth occupied, which may sound silly, but for many folks, it's an avoidance thing: If your mouth is being occupied by a nearly-nil-calorie coffee, that keeps it away from a zillion-calorie alternative.

I Accept Cheating as a Reward, Not a Sin.

I could make the argument that one of the reasons I struggled so much during my life is because of the way I viewed so-called bad foods that taste great. I'd vow to eat right, deviate, then throw my hands up in defeat and say, "Might as well suck up some ravioli." Once I learned, and really felt, that I could go down the dark alley of eating every once in a while, I'd emerge on the other side okay. After a while, because I found substitutions that satisfied cravings, I discovered that I didn't need cheat meals or snacks as much. I didn't banish them completely, because I believe that bad food can bring pleasure, even if it's just temporary, and if you eat well 90 percent of the time, then you don't have to feel guilty about the occasional chicken-parm sandwich. Some research indicates that cheating can help not only psychologically (a mental reward for those who are on restrictive diets), but also because it can cause boosts of the hormone leptin, which can increase metabolism and control appetite. The danger, as Attia pointed out, is keeping that 10 percent (or thereabouts) at 10 percent. Can you keep it from sliding so that a cheat meal turns into a cheat day turns into a cheat weekend turns into "Thursday is part of the weekend, right?" This is perhaps the toughest task of all when trying to eat well, but I'd argue that if the other truths I've outlined here are working, it makes it easier for this one to work, too. How did I do it? I guess my approach worked like this: I stopped thinking I had to follow a rule (such as "I get only one cheat meal a week") and started telling myself that I would try to win the week—"Get through the week eating well, and you can give yourself some flexibility come the weekend." When I won the week, I didn't have as much desire to ravage through the weekend with wing sauce on my chin. Because of that, when I did feel an urge to be a little bad, I indulged. Without the guilt. Without having to make it a monster portion. Without having the snowball consequences of two slices of pizza leading to a whole box.

Some of my current eating approach revolves around choosing the right kinds of foods, but some involves the method in which I eat them. After years of trial and denial, I realized that in order not only to be successful at how I wanted my body to be, but also to indulge in some of the pleasures of eating, I had to work on both—the what as well as the how. Eat healthy foods most of the time, but be aware that how you deliver them to yourself—be it by counting calories or intermittently fasting or declaring a cheat meal every week or some other method—can be just as important. Smart nutrition, especially when just starting out or making a big change in the way you approach it, also requires smart action—action that you can sustain, action that gives you some wiggle room if you want, and action that allows you to match your personality to your pleasures—a principle that holds true for exercise as well.

8. PERSPIRATION

Truth: Playing Hard Never Feels Like Hard Work

Several years ago, sick of my creeping weight levels, I finally signed up to work with a trainer. I didn't call him a trainer, because that would have been admitting I needed help. No, I didn't need help, even though I topped 260 at the time; I wanted to improve my basketball skills, so I needed a sports performance coach, and that's what I called him. I met Jeff Plasschaert twice a week for a while, and I immediately loved his approach. Even though I moved more like a cement truck than a motorcycle, Jeff treated me like an athlete. He didn't just assign me vanilla exercises and watch me perform them, in the way you'd imagine some trainers worked. He always created something new for me to try, to challenge myself, and he put together programs that *real* athletes would have done.

Things he made me do: Push heavy weights across the floor in a low bear crawl (a real glute burner). Get into push-up position and walk my hands around in a circle, pausing to do push-ups at three o'clock, six, nine, and twelve (a real shoulder burner). Chase after a tennis ball like a Labrador and then decelerate before I ran into a wall (a real ego burner). One time, during a pool workout, he handed me a twenty-five-pound weight plate and told me to hold it against my chest and swim to the side. I sank. He laughed. I still work with Jeff off and on, but I will always be grateful to him not only for pushing me hard by changing up my workout every time, but also for introducing me to tire flipping.

One day, he took me outside and showed me the stash of tires he had—truck tires, tractor tires, small tires, big tires. We used them to do all kinds of moves. I flipped them. I slammed them with sledgehammers. I jumped on them. And I got hooked. The scrap heap of rubber became my favorite new piece of exercise equipment, so much so that now I have a 40-pound forklift tire, a 140-pound truck tire, and a crane tire that, from the best I can tell, weighs about 750 pounds.

One day, during a contest with two buddies to see how many flips we each could do in two minutes, I decided to go crazy. (I had lost the rest of the mini-competitions that day.) Gas pedal, all out, just go. When I finished my flips, the worst headache I'd ever had started pinballing through my skull—to the point where I thought, "Holy hell, my brain is going to explode all over the yard because why? Because I wanted to get a few more flips than my friends?" The pain downgraded from sharp to dull after a few minutes, but lingered for the next day or so. (My Internet searching scared me enough to get tested, to rule out some kind of aneurysm, and all turned out fine. It was just an exertion headache, likely caused by all the crazy changes my blood vessels were going through as my head bobbed up and down for those two minutes. I also learned that some people experience these exertion headaches during orgasm.)

Was besting my friends worth the scare? Of course not, but as someone who has never experienced what it feels like to go past the point you think you're able to go athletically, I found it liberating, because it was one of the few times when I allowed my mind to out-talk my body—to tell it, "Enough, you soft cookie-chewing sloth. Go hard."

Turns out, *go hard* may just be the two most important words for any exercise plan.

"You Can't Out-Train Your Diet"

For most of my adulthood, I've exercised regularly, even when I've weighed my heaviest. In fact, there are only a few stretches in my life—once when I was overwhelmed with some work projects and once when I pulled my back—when I remember skipping workouts for more than a couple of weeks. During that stretch, I went to the doc's office for a physical, at a time when my weight was up (in the low 260s) and he asked me if I exercised.

"I yo-yo," I said, trying to make the clear-to-me metaphor between yo-yo dieting and off-and-on exercise.

He paused.

Then he raised his eyebrow. "Like yo-yo?" he asked, playing out the action of a child playing with the toy.

Geezuz. How fat am I that he thinks that I think yo-yo would count as exercise?

After I clarified that I had been off a routine for a bit, he went about his rubber-glove business, and I was on my way. (I soon changed doctors.) But that small stretch in my life was really the only time I can remember taking "off" from working out. Sometimes, I glided through—just going through the motions, rationalizing that if I was at the gym, that counted (but it didn't).

I love sweating and lifting and playing, and I feel like I've tried just about every kind of exercise out there—but not in the "tried every diet" kind of way. One of the foundations of fitness is challenging your body differently. As soon as your body adapts to one form of exercise, that's when the fitness gains (and weight loss) stop, so continually changing a routine, to me, feels like a crucial element.

I've tried step class, Pilates, and yoga. I tried aqua aerobics. I've done boot camps. I love spinning. I run, swim, and mountain bike. I love my old-man basketball games. I lift weights. I've logged time on rowing machines, stair climbers, treadmills, and elliptical machines. I once took boxing lessons (which, to this day, remains one of the best and hardest workouts I've ever done, because it works all your muscles, your cardio system, and the I'm-about-to-get-rocked fight-or-flight response). I've worked by myself and in groups. And I can't count the number of times my nipples have bled from chafing while I ran. I like to exercise, I like virtually all forms, and I think all of them have a place in someone's life. Do what you love, and you'll see benefits.

My laundry list begs the obvious question: If you've tried all that, and if you are consistent with your workouts, why have you struggled so much with your weight? The answer comes in the form of what my former *Men's Health* colleague Adam Campbell has said many times: "You can't out-train your diet." That, before any discussion about exercise effectiveness, is *it*. Unless you're logging Michael Phelpsian hours in whatever activity you're doing or have a metabolism as hot as the sun's surface, you're likely not going to be able to burn enough calories to keep up with crappy diets and crappy foods. But what happens if you do get the food part together? What's the best way to train?

It appears that some activities are more effective than others, but I also believe that *anything* can work. So if you like one particular exercise, and that's what you'll stick with, then that's what you should do. It may just take a little longer for the effects to kick in. Plenty of people have lost a lot of weight only running or only swimming or even only walking, which is why one of the first things Dr. Michael Roizen prescribes in his weight-loss programs is thirty minutes of walking every day (it's about the movement, the commitment, and the consistency). All physical activities burn calories, and over time, combined with a healthy diet, you can lose weight (or maintain a good weight) with any exercise.

If we're talking about what's best in terms of sheer effectiveness at burning fat the fastest, changing your shape, and getting into the best condition of your life, your exercise approach should include two things: adding muscle and adding intensity.

Muscle: For Everyone

It used to be that a lot of people looked at muscle with the same disdain with which they looked at, say, the aftereffects of cabbage. That's likely because people thought that if you tried to build muscle, you'd end up looking like a 1970s Schwarzenegger. That mind-set has shifted some, in that more and more weight-loss prescriptions call for the addition of muscle to help men and women with fat burning.

Skeletal muscle tissues (as opposed to cardiac muscle tissue or smooth muscle tissue that's associated with the function of organs) have cells different from other cells in the body. They're large and they run the length of the entire muscle. Because of that, muscle cells are one of the few in the body that have multiple nuclei inside them. The reason they need to be long is because of the way they work. To generate force—to help you walk, run, lift, live, or any other verb that puts you in motion—the cells shorten, generating a "pull," and then relax, letting the "pull" go. Muscles also have different fibers (another name for cells) that do different jobs. The small and skinny red fibers are "slow-twitch" fibers; they're what give us muscular endurance (the ability to hold our head on our necks all day when we work, or run 26.2 miles if we so choose). They use oxygen to make energy and can work all damn day, but they don't generate much power. The larger, white fibers in the muscle, the "fast-twitch" fibers, are what generate more tension and more force. They don't rely as heavily on oxygen, but rather on other energy sources in the body that are used up quickly, so they can be used for only short amounts of time. They're the ones used by bodybuilders and sprinters, and by all of us to get up from the couch: the folks who need their bodies to generate a lot of force in a short time.

We also know that muscle cells, just like fat cells, have plasticity (meaning that they can get bigger and smaller) and that they can adapt depending on how you use them, said Joslyn Ahlgren, PhD, the anatomy and physiology professor from the University of Florida. So you can take your in-between cells (ones that don't fall into either category) and develop them to be smaller or larger, depending on what you do with them.

Most people look at skeletal muscle as simply being used to help the body move, but it serves other purposes, such as maintaining body heat. (As cells break down energy molecules to fuel muscle contractions, some of that energy is lost as heat. That heat accumulates in cells; producing sweat is one of the ways we can lose some of that heat, and thus get cool, as it's transferred to Big Tony's sweat droplets on the gym machines.) Yes, muscles help us perform daily functions, but the role they play in weight loss is to help you chew up fat. "I've been telling people from day one, you can't just do cardio and expect to change your body composition. You need to enhance your lean muscle mass," Ahlgren said.

Here's why: Your muscle cells are highly metabolic; it takes a lot more energy to maintain muscle than it does to maintain fat. So when you add muscle mass, more calories get burned up trying to maintain that muscle than would go toward maintaining fat. "If I can have more cells in my body with that metabolic rate, I will have a higher metabolic rate," Ahlgren said. "And even just sitting here, I will use more calories at rest than I would otherwise."

When you eat food, your body breaks down those nutrients, absorbs them, and then delivers them throughout your body to use for energy to power those organs and systems. If you eat too much, your body holds on to those calories to give you a steady feed—kind of like an IV drip throughout the day. But if you eat more than can be used, you just end up storing it through fat.

When you add muscle, your body can take from the hoard you've stashed and use that to feed those muscles. Inside your fat cells (which never go away, by the way; they just shrink if you lose weight), fat is stored mostly in the form of triglycerides—that's what's pulled from your fat cells when your body needs the energy elsewhere. With muscle, your body wants to pull that energy and feed the muscle. Look at what happens when you have a limb in a cast. The body says, "What the heck. I'm not using this muscle, so I'm not wasting energy on going to something that's not being used," so the muscle shrinks. The opposite reaction is in effect when you build muscle. Your body needs to feed that muscle, so it pulls energy (which would otherwise become fat) to do so.

In addition, resistance training improves insulin sensitivity, meaning that your body won't overreact every time you binge. "What you can learn from lean and muscular people is not that they can eat whatever they want and not put on fat," said Adam Bornstein. "It's the opposite. Because they have less fat and more muscle, it gives them greater freedom to eat what they want because the calories they take in won't have the same impact on their hormones and insulin as someone with a much higher percentage of body fat."

Amp Up Your Intensity Levels

For a long time, low-impact, long-duration cardiovascular exercise was prescribed for weight loss. That's because when cells were asked for energy for a longer amount of time, it required them to burn fat rather than carbohydrates, Ahlgren said, so if that's what the body wanted to burn, then heck, yeah, that's what will burn fat. Back then, researchers didn't consider the metabolic demand that muscles have, that muscles help deplete fat stores.

We also didn't consider the effect that shorter-duration, higher-intensity workouts would have on our calorie-burning systems. With those brief, high-intensity sessions—think twenty minutes, alternating between all out and rest, rather than an hour at the same steady speed—your body relies on readily available carbohydrate stores for energy, much more so than that needed at low intensity. At some point, the intensity of that exercise will demand that you burn fat as well. "So with a combination of resistance training and intense exercise, you're setting yourself up for a high metabolism, just to maintain a normal, healthy body," Ahlgren said.

High-intensity interval training has a lot of upsides: It's effective and it's efficient—you can get benefits with twenty minutes of work as opposed to an hour—but it also has two very real roadblocks: First, people need to be ready for it in a way they wouldn't necessarily have to, say, go for an hour-long walk every day. That is, most of us can just start a walking program, but starting a high-intensity program should have a doctor's approval. Second, a lot of people simply don't tolerate high-intensity sessions psychologically. Ask someone if they'd rather go five minutes longer doing what they're doing or go much more intensely for a shorter period of time, and they'll usually choose duration over intensity. (Like anything, tolerance to intensity is something you can train for.)

In a 2012 review of studies looking at high-intensity interval training published in the *Journal of Physiology*, researchers concluded that this type of training has both cardiovascular and muscular health benefits. Though there's not a significant amount of research that points to weight loss as one of its benefits, small studies show that this kind of training does aid the chemical processes associated with fat burning, in that it helps you burn calories even after you've stopped the activity.

This is where the gains (and losses) happen: High-intensity workouts change body shapes and sizes (they've done so for me). Even if it appears that some kind of combination of resistance exercise and high-intensity workouts should be staples of workout programs, it doesn't matter what's most effective if you don't exercise at all, meaning that just starting has to be the first step for some people.

When we're dealing with people who need to lose weight, the first question may not be which is the right exercise to do, said Alex Hutchinson, PhD, author of the book *Which Comes First, Cardio or Weights?*. "All of that is noise on top of the signal. Are you exercising or are you not exercising? That's the question that matters."

Everyone starts with good intentions, said Hutchinson, who believes in modest goals that end up producing results. Most people overestimate what they can do in the short term and underestimate what they can do in the long term. "What's the right exercise?" Hutchinson said. "Something you're going to be interested in and tolerate doing, and will not take a big mental effort to will yourself to do. When people ask about [specific] exercise or diet programs, are they magic bullets? No. There are a billion ways of exercising and a few ways of eating well, which all produce good results. And whichever particular environment gets people fired up, fantastic. So the answer isn't to the question 'What should you do?' It's 'What are you willing to do and what are you interested in doing?'"

The reason those seem to be the correct questions seems to be that so many other factors play a role in how our bodies function—what we eat, how much we move throughout the rest of the day, the quality and quantity of the sleep we get, genetic issues—so that finding the one set plan that will work for everyone is a reflection not so much of the plan itself, but of the body (and personality) doing it. Even Hutchinson, happily a runner (and a darn fast one at that, having run a 2:44 marathon), knows he has to make adjustments.

"Over the last few years, the science of fitness has shown that variety is really important, that to be maximally healthy you can't just exercise the same way all the time. To slow down the inevitable loss of health, I realize I need to do more full-body exercise—circuit training, rock climbing," said Hutchinson, who even changed up his regular running routine to include two days of resistance training. "From a health and longevity perspective, there's no question that this is important. Running doesn't prepare you to get up from a very soft couch when you're seventy-five or stay balanced on an icy surface."

So the most effective formula for fat loss would include some weight training and some higher-intensity exercise. An important note: One of the reasons people avoid lifting weights is because of the fear of bulking up and adding pounds to the scale; while that can happen with many other variables, including eating more, what happens more often is that your body composition will shift—your percentage of weight shifts to one of more muscle and less fat. And you end up burning *more* calories, because it takes your body more calories to maintain muscle than it does to maintain fat.

I can tell you that anytime I've lost a significant number of pounds, weight training (three times a week) and higher-intensity workouts of running, spinning class, or tire flipping were part of the mix. Most times when I trained for endurance events doing primarily steady-state exercise, I either hit a plateau or gained some weight. That's not an indictment of cardiovascular exercise itself. (After all, lots of runners are lean.) Steady-state activity does burn calories, work your cardiovascular system, and provide a million other stress-relieving, mood-boosting, and body-improving benefits. The reason may have more to do with hunger and appetite in relationship to exercise, especially long bouts of cardiovascular work. Though some research points to decreases in appetite after exercise, there's no question that the opposite holds true for many people—and that many of us use rationalization to justify post-exercise eating (e.g., "I ran for an hour; I'll have the foot-long steak sandwich"). And that reinforces a fundamental principle of exercise, along with my other truths: No one thing can be the answer; all things should work in concert to improve your chances of being successful.

Three Essential Elements of Exercise

The answer for most people lies not in specific plans or programs, but in stepping back with some overarching philosophies about what you want for your workouts. Looking at your tastes in these three areas can help you determine what forms of exercise you want to use:

- **Goal setting:** Especially important for endurance-oriented people, setting goals, and then picking the process about how to get there, provides the foundation.
- **Variety:** Variety means ideally mixing in some kind of muscle training and higher-intensity cardio, not only for the physiological benefits, but also the psychological ones. This doesn't mean you have to change up everything you do. Even if you like one particular activity (i.e., weight training or running), mixing up workouts, duration, intensities, and movements adds an element of variety that keeps you from getting bored.
- **Play:** Create an environment that makes exercise feel more like recess than a routine, to encourage you to

keep it up. You do it because you like doing it, not because you feel you have to. A reward in itself, not a
chore to be done with.

Sometimes, it may seem that these three things compete
against one another (having a process versus having a sense of
play), but all three can work together. When they do, it may just
create the ideal environment for fighting fat.

This is likely one of the reasons we've seen an explosion in the
area of CrossFit, a system that combines high-intensity strength
moves with high-intensity cardio work, where workouts change
up all the time and participants compete against themselves and
each other to better their marks. To get a sense of what a CrossFit
workout looks like, you may have to do a certain number of pull-
ups, Olympic-style barbell lifts, and sprints in as quick a time as
you can. There's no question that CrossFit has exploded in
popularity—there are more than ten thousand CrossFit-branded
gyms—and if you look at the bodies of the top CrossFitters,
you'll see they fit the definition of lean and strong. That's not to
say that CrossFit doesn't have its critics. *Gawker* featured a piece
called "The Problem(s) with CrossFit" and *Outside* magazine
asked, "Is CrossFit Killing Us?" The main argument against
CrossFit (besides the high cost of belonging to these gyms) is
that people not properly trained in form (especially with the
Olympic lifts with heavy weights) are more prone to injuries.
That's because of the nature of CrossFit: You're encouraged to lift
heavier weights in rapid-fire repetitions. Supporters would argue
that, hey, if you have the right form, CrossFit is no more dangerous than any other mode of exercise. User error, not activity
error.

One small study in the *Journal of Conditioning and Strength Research* found that men doing a CrossFit-based power-training program dropped from 22 percent body fat to 18 percent in ten weeks, while women went from almost 27 percent to 23 percent. Another study in the same journal found that while CrossFitters did make significant fitness gains, 16 percent dropped out of the activity because of overuse or an injury. A London study—one whose authors said they believed was the first to examine injury rates among CrossFitters—pointed out that injury rates among participants were no different from those who participated in sports such as gymnastics and power lifting, and were lower than injury rates in contact sports. All this is to say, yes, it can be really effective. And yes, like any other sport, you can get hurt doing it, especially if you don't take precautions and do it safely.

I have not tried CrossFit per se, so I can't tell you firsthand what I think about it. (Why? Big boy scared of pull-ups, even the modified kind that CrossFitters do, in which they use their core and legs to let momentum help them up.) I have known people who've loved it and those who swear it caused them injury. But I believe the reason it's not only popular but also effective is because it employs all the elements that make for an effective body-changing program—emphasizing muscle, intensity, variety, competition, and fun.

What's Your Definition of Fun?

My second source of inspiration for my tire-flipping workouts came from an assignment I had for *Men's Health*: watching the training sessions of Martin Rooney, a former U.S. bobsled team member who made his name training all kinds of athletes, but mainly different kinds of mixed martial arts fighters. Rooney, with a black belt in judo and a purple belt in Brazilian jiujitsu, exudes energy, confidence, and a let's-tackle-this-together aura that makes you want to drop thirty pounds on the spot and then go lift a tank over your head.

When I went to watch him train a group of fighters, I had two emotions. I was excited to see him in action, because I had heard many good things about him and was curious about the oxymoron of a "fun-loving fighter," but I was also upset because I was so badly out of shape that I was embarrassed to ask him if I could join the group and do the workout with them (not that I could keep up with elite fighters, but as part of my job, I wanted to try to feel what they felt). So I didn't even ask if I could join in.

Rooney took the group, a mix of younger and older fighters, through a warm-up that would have left most people done for the day. In that warm-up and some subsequent moves, he built a crescendo toward his signature series, a group of moves called the Hurricane, which works like this: Rooney picks five stations, and each athlete goes at it at a particular one for one minute, as hard as he can, and then moves to the next station immediately. You do all five in a row, then rest. Then you do them again. And again. Fifteen minutes of work may not sound like much, but when you're going as hard as you can in such things as sledgehammer hits on a tire or carrying a hundred-plus-pound bag of sand or pushing a weight-packed sled across the floor, it can feel as if you're trying to lift an elephant by its trunk. When the group was finished, they weren't finished. They went across the room and did sprints—with Rooney right there running with them.

Rooney's goal, then, was to prepare his athletes to withstand the intense brutality of being in a ring where another man is trying to pound your every fiber. It struck me that all three elements (goal setting, variety, and play) were working together: The athletes had a goal (in most cases, their next fight). They had variety within the workout (that's the nature of Hurricanes, different moves all strung together). And in many cases, even though they were pushing themselves hard, the very design of the workout appeared upbeat, fast, fun—that is, like play. They fed off each other, they pushed each other, they competed. In a way, they didn't even need to *think* about the intensity.

In those few days, I talked to Rooney a lot—mostly about his Training for Warriors philosophy and how what he does isn't about getting everyone prepared for a cage fight, but rather getting them to take on the rigors they'll come across in their lives.

"The warrior is process-oriented, not outcome-oriented," he told me. "They have to train like, when the fight gets here, they gotta know that, win or lose, they know they did what they could. So many people live this unfulfilled life. They're always so focused on the outcome and then when it doesn't happen the way they want, then they think everything was a waste along the way. But, man, if you've done your best, regardless of the outcome, you're going to be okay with it. I call it the warrior test. If you wake up in the morning and ask yourself, 'Hey, what am I going to do today?' and at the end of the day, you ask, 'What did I do today?' If you fail that test enough days in a row, you're not going to be something. If you pass that test enough days in a row, I guarantee you can't imagine what you can accomplish in a hundred days, let alone years."

One of the ways I like to look at this area of fitness is the way I look at college. As a professor, I may have a student for one, maybe two classes throughout his entire college career. What I say or teach or critique may help him in his career, or it may be forgotten the moment he leaves the room, if he even heard it in the first place. But no matter what or how much (or how little) is absorbed, the whole point of most college majors is for the student to get a wide variety of experiences and instruction and information—and to use what he does need and filter out what he doesn't. The realm of training is like that. We should take bits and pieces from a variety of sources and figure out what works best for us. So on the one hand, I'll see the power of goal setting— the mechanism that drives many people forward to make good decisions, to stick to a plan, to stay locked on target, and to change their bodies. On the other hand, I'll meet people like Rob Corbett.

Corbett contacted me a few years ago about a book project he was working on called *Just Groove*. I've never met him in person, and I've talked with him on the phone only a few times over the years, but after reading his work, I feel like I know him better than I know some of the people with offices in the same hallway as mine. The backstory: Years ago, as a stressed-out writer for MTV, Corbett used music to pull himself out of a depression and a bad path in his personal life. After chasing happiness in all the wrong ways as a young man, he started jamming on instruments at home every night after work as a stress release, and realized he could feel better every day just by grooving in simple ways.

As he started researching his book, he learned that music is in our DNA. (Just watch a baby groove to it.) So he put on his headphones and started grooving around the house for fun exercise. (Note: Corbett says the word *dance* has become so loaded in our culture that it intimidates most men, keeping them from just moving to music for fun, because they think "dancing" requires choreography and dance classes and pressure and other stress-inducers that make the average guy say, "Nope, I can't dance.") Soon Corbett switched gears from writing a book to reinventing an industry. He realized that over the past forty years (specifically, since the sneaker boom), we've become the first people in history whose feet are impeded by unnatural rubber traction all the time (meaning we can't spin and twist the way we could with the natural foot-twisting motions of the rock 'n' roll revolution or the 1970s era of disco and *Soul Train*, the last era when guys still wore natural leather-soled shoes out to clubs before rubber soles took over our culture). Eventually, Corbett created a sneaker company, the Groove Revolution (GRV shoes), "the world's first sneakers with natural leather soles that unlock your natural soul."

One of the big things that Corbett noticed when he started grooving for fun is that it had a dramatic effect on his body and his energy. That's when he saw grooving as having incredible potential for people desperate to find an exercise method they could enjoy (instead of dread, for those who dreaded traditional modes of exercise). Corbett even went to USC's sports science lab to test the caloric burn involved in using his shoes with various exercise movements, and he got in the best shape of his life—by just grooving. No goals, no programs, no regimens, no reps, no sets, no weight lifting, no running, no equipment, no pressure. Just fun. From doing something he loved—and wanting to do it over and over because of the way it made him feel (which is Doug Newburg's whole point about the skill of feel, right?).

If you were to ask both Corbett and Rooney what works when it comes to exercise, they couldn't be on more opposite ends of the continuum. But they're both right—and using the two approaches is probably the mix that works for most people: having the discipline and hunger to be consistent and push yourself, but having the free spirit to find something that gets you moving every day for the fun of it.

This is probably why my favorite exercise session of the week is my Friday session with friends. In it, we run, we flip, we lift, we sprint, we throw balls, we use sledgehammers, we change it up all the time. It's typically my hardest workout of the week, but it never feels like a chore.

The conclusion isn't that you have to do something that feels as if it's laced with testosterone (even though just as many women come to my tire-flipping workouts as men, and a reported 60 percent of CrossFitters are women). The conclusion is that those who want to lose weight should be doing a few weight workouts a week, be it with dumbbells, machines, bands, or even knocking out some push-ups and bodyweight squats. You won't Hulk up doing so, but you will add fat-burning muscle. Whatever other activity you do, you should make a point to push yourself past your comfort level. That goes for spinning class, Zumba, running, even walking (e.g., a thirty-minute walk in which you alternate periods of fast walking with a moderate pace is better than thirty minutes of moderate pace only). And if you can do it all without feeling it's the worst thing you've ever put your body through, you've won the battle.

A few days before my second Tough Mudder event (an obstacle-course I run with friends that I'll talk more about in a few chapters), I tweeted that I was looking forward to the day and to doing these things: "Run, jump, crawl, fall, freeze, sweat, freak, climb, swim, slog, push, laugh, HAMMER, triumph."

My friend Doug Newburg, the performance coach, immediately e-mailed me, pointing out that my tweet was revealing: The process was more meaningful than the goal.

"Your tweet is awesome because they are all words that elicit a feel when you think about them. None of them are about winning or performing," he wrote. "That's the whole point."

PART 3

Your Best Size: Getting the Body You Want—for Good

9. DEDICATION

Truth: Authentic Progress Happens When No One's Watching

I met Christine Dougherty because of tacos.

Christine had gained weight after her teenage years the way many of us do—as office jobs and fried foods catch up to us. When she made eating changes, she lost more than fifty pounds. Because she ate some of her meals at Taco Bell, she became the spokesperson for Taco Bell's Drive-Thru Diet. This fact meant that I, a one-time regular consumer of their now defunct chili-cheese burrito, had to talk to her. A few years back, I interviewed Christine about her diet, her weight loss, and running the New York City Marathon the same year as I did. Initially, to lose the weight, she counted calories and changed most of her food choices to healthy ones. She lost the weight slowly (over more than two years), which she believes is what has prevented her from yo-yoing or regaining a lot of weight.

Her cholesterol dropped, and a mysterious pain that used to creep up her right side from time to time disappeared. She also got rid of any symptoms from irritable bowel syndrome. But she wasn't entirely satisfied. Christine, who is five foot four and dropped from 154 to 105 pounds, was doing a lot of cardiovascular work. "I was thin and skinny," she said, "but I didn't have muscles. I didn't feel strong."

Now, years later and even though she had much weight-loss success, Christine has changed her approach to eating and exercise. She's focused on eating muscle-building protein, healthy fats, fiber, and vegetables, and she's started doing more strength training. The result: Her body changed. She stayed petite (although she did gain some weight back because of the muscle), but morphed from looking thin to looking (and being) strong. (I can attest to this, because Christine joined our Tough Mudder team one year and crushed the monkey bars and all the other obstacles in our way.)

The real result, the deeper result: She's happy. She rarely gets sick. She's in a good mood. She's confident.

Best of all, she said, it doesn't take a lot of work to maintain what she's done, because she likes what she's doing. She exercises for shorter amounts of time than she did while doing a lot of cardio training, and she really focuses on eating the foods she likes: eggs, oatmeal, broccoli, hummus, asparagus, black beans, avocado, brown rice, and protein shakes. If she wants to indulge in something that's not healthy, she limits it to small portions.

"Even if I could maintain my weight loss without eating better or working out, like genetically blessed people, I would still eat better and work out because it makes me healthier, and I feel awesome," she said. "I get to enjoy life more."

So many of us (me included) chase the number, chase the weight. But when the chase is about something bigger, it's easier for all the factors to fall into place. I used to think that the battle was about being a bulldozer when it came to making choices, outmuscling the bad foods in the pantry or at restaurants (*I am stronger than your evil ingredients!*), but I've come to learn that for all the pieces to fall into place, it's more about dedication. It's quieter than what we typically think of as determination. Christine doesn't have to struggle to reach her goal (that's not to say she doesn't work out hard or have challenges), but it doesn't feel like a struggle, because she found the answers that not only work, but that she *likes*.

As my friend Doug would say, Christine feels good because she's living by feel.

Dedicated and Determined to Do What?

When I complained on Twitter about a few injury aches I was having during my training, Lonnie St John asked if I needed to call the "waaaaaaaaaaaahbulance."

A taunt. A friendly taunt, but a taunt nonetheless. Immediately, I liked the guy. He was basically telling me to suck it up, stop complaining, and do the work I needed to do to achieve my goals. I soon learned that Lonnie had earned the right to say such things. Very early on in our acquaintance, when I woke up and checked my Twitter feed at around 7:00 a.m., I saw that Lonnie had posted that he was at the gym to do his weekday runs. He lived three time zones behind me. "Holy hell," I thought, "this man is focused."

We interacted virtually more and more over time, and soon he blew me away with his story: In a period of eighteen months, Lonnie went from weighing more than three hundred pounds to trying to qualify for the Boston Marathon.

Lonnie's how-I-got-fat story: He was raised by a single mom, and his father figure was an uncle who weighed four hundred-some pounds. What Lonnie remembers most was that his uncle's name was Dooner, and everyone called Lonnie "Dooner Junior" because of his weight. "I knew why they were saying that, but I look back now and think, 'That's not very nice,'" he said. His family ate a lot of processed foods, and the concept of portion control was off-limits. "I remember my mom played softball, and after every practice, we would go have pizza at our favorite pizza place, and we would eat until we were stuffed, wait a half hour, go to the bathroom, come back, and eat some more," he said.

Lonnie was overweight his whole life, went through a couple of periods when the family decided everyone would diet, and he had some successes. He reached 276 pounds in high school, lost some weight, joined the military, and then was discharged after two years because he had ballooned back up to 250. Stationed in Germany, nine time zones away from home, he'd return to his house after duty and have a bag of caramels and a six-pack of Cherry Coke for dinner. Lonnie reached his top known weight of 317 (though he suspects he could have been close to 340), and that's when he started to change: He lost it through calorie counting and running. He had always liked sports, especially basketball, but few people are interested in a three-hundred-pound guy who can shoot. Running allowed him a chance to compete with himself. "The competitive drive was 'Can I be better today than I was yesterday?'" Lonnie started hitting his stride by running about fifteen to twenty miles per week, and the weight kept dropping. He remembered the turning point: He was in a local running store and he ran into a guy "more fit than I could ever imagine to be," whom he knew from the gym. "He recognized me—he never paid attention to me at the gym—and he told the clerk, 'This guy'—meaning me—'is an awesome runner,'" Lonnie said.

Lonnie started to feed off not pepperoni, but the positive feedback he received, especially from his wife, Roni, and his friends. He also took a few hits of negative feedback. One time, a former school friend who saw he was having success running, wrote this to Lonnie: "You think you're hot shit with all your running. You're still just a fat ass. I don't run at all and would kick your ass in a race." Lonnie posted this on his Facebook timeline and challenged his former friend to a race. He never heard from him again.

"Haters are motivators," Lonnie told me. "My trainer asked me how he should approach me when I have a failure, so I can best bounce back. I said, 'Don't coddle me. If you want to get me going, get me pissed off. That's when I'll respond. Being nice to me makes me comfortable and I won't get results that way.' I prefer jeers to cheers."

When he hit 250 pounds, Lonnie got hooked and wanted to see how far he could take this. He started racing, and even challenged his daughter, who runs cross-country, to a race. He did his first 5K in thirty-five minutes, then did his next in twenty-eight minutes. Then his times kept getting faster and faster, to the point where he was winning his age groups and finishing in the lead pack of a local race—his best time is a 21:05, which averages to a 6:47 mile, and he plans to drop to under 20:00. He then ran his best half marathon in 1:36:15. This made him decide he wanted to run a marathon, and not just run it, but qualify for Boston—which meant he'd have to run a 3:15. For a guy who weighed more than three hundred pounds not too long before, that seemed damn near impossible. Turns out, Lonnie completed his first marathon but was dehydrated and finished slower than he wanted, not qualifying for Boston. That didn't matter, I'd argue. What did is that he still focused on trying to qualify for Boston, beat his other race times, and did things in running that he never dreamed he could do when he weighed more than three hundred pounds.

Lonnie said the reason he's so dedicated to his mission is because he refuses to do what he's done in the past with weight-loss efforts: give up. "Stopping is the only true failure in life," he said. "I don't want this to be another example of me just giving up because it got hard. I have people reaching out to me regularly, reminding me that I'm not in this alone and how I encourage them just by showing up. I may have days where I want to quit on myself, but I sure as hell can't quit on them."

In the pop culture sense, determination is about rah-rah, about grit, about locker room speeches, about running through walls. The word connotes power, persistence, sweat, will. In more psychological terms, determination is woven into the concept of motivation (and those three psychological needs outlined in chapter 6: autonomy, relatedness, and competence) and is the thing that drives people toward their goals.

Leslie Podlog, PhD, an assistant professor of exercise and sport science at the University of Utah who studies and teaches about the intersection of psychology and sports behavior, told me that a better way to think about determination is as "energy." What do you want to direct your energy toward (i.e., what is the goal)? How energized are you to meet that goal? And how much can you persist in the face of setbacks? Podlog, who entered this field as a former wrestler who was injured so much that he spent more time in physical therapy than on the mat, mainly studies injured athletes and how they cope with those energy levels. While not exactly a similar scenario, there are parallels between the injured athlete and those trying to lose weight. Both may have experienced some previous success, they got derailed (whether by injury or gaining weight), and they're seeing if they have the determination to make it back to where they once were (or where they'd like to be). "For the athlete with an injury," Podlog said, "the first question is 'Is this something I want to continue doing and how much effort and energy persistence am I willing to put forward in achieving that goal?'" Podlog said that in some research he's done, it seems that the psychological needs of competence and relatedness seem to be more important than autonomy. For athletes, they want a sense of control in deciding to undertake their rehab, but once that decision has been made, they release the control and want to be in the hands of others who can help them. This makes sense. Once I've made the decision to come back, give me the program, and I'll follow it. This is the same way a diet works for so many: You say you want to take control and lose weight, but then want the prescription for what to do. The step that might be missing for some dieters, though, is that in order to work, that element of relatedness needs to be present—to help with the concept of energy to work around setbacks. Without that community to prod you forward, to help you maintain energy when nobody is looking, you fall back into your old habits. In the case of injured athletes on a rehab program, there's a built-in community, be it in the form of a team, coaches, physical therapists, or docs. What makes it most difficult is that this period— whether it's spent in rehab or trying to losing weight—is filled with tension.

"The nature of transition is uncertainty, and uncertainty is an aversive state," Podlog said. "When there's no certainty, there's a lack of control, and that creates anxiety."

Which is why there's so much emphasis on setting goals. (The research indicates that the most effective goals must be specific, challenging but reasonable, time-based, and must have an element through which people can evaluate whether the goal has been achieved.)

This is why Lonnie's story moves me so much. Here's a guy who looked more like a sumo wrestler than a marathoner and who's had so much success losing weight *and* improving athletic performance in such a short period of time that I'm blown away by his dedication. He makes no excuses, just does the work, on good days and bad, and he changed his body—and really his life. I look at him and think, "Wow." I also look at him and think, "How?"—as in, "How in the world could he get so damn fast and do it so damn fast, while I've been sitting here spinning my wheels for years, for decades?"

Why Failure to Reach a Goal Isn't Failure

Soon after my molasses marathon, I took a step back and reevaluated where I was. Instead of trying to take on a bigger challenge, I decided I needed to take on a faster one. I needed to get leaner, stronger, quicker, so in my blog, I declared that my next goal would not be some epic event. Instead, I would get back to the basics, and try to run a sub-thirty-minute 5K. For many runners, this time would feel like a crawl, but for me and a lot of other folks, this number actually serves as a symbolic entryway—from the back of the back up toward the middle. To get under thirty minutes, I told myself, would make me feel as if I made some progress. (My previous best time hung around thirty-four minutes, I believe.) On my first attempt out, without much speed-specific training, I finished somewhere around the thirty-three-minute mark. This race served as the baseline for where I was, and what I needed to do. On my next attempt, I hit a 30:19.

Sean Limon, my friend and the man who convinced me to sign up for an Ironman, likes to quote Yoda when taking on challenges such as these: "Do or do not. There is no try." I've attempted to have philosophical discussions with Sean about Yoda. My argument: There are some things in life you can try as hard as you can to do and you still may not be able to do them. Sean didn't accept that. Do or do not, he maintained.

I had targeted an April race a few weeks away for my next attempt to go sub-thirty. That race came at the peak heat of a Florida day, at around 5:00 p.m. It was run on a golf course (not the faster blacktop), and the air was still smoky from wildfires in the area. (Also, I had had a few pieces of the kids' Easter candy in the few days leading up to the race.) I tweeted about the obstacles, and a few people replied with "no excuses" comments. Deep down, I could feel I wasn't going to hit sub-thirty that day.

When the gun went off, I ran hard, but when I checked my watch, I could tell I was already behind my target pace a half mile in, and knew I wouldn't make the time. I was right. I finished slightly over thirty-two minutes and immediately tweeted this:

"Sub-thirty fail. Eff Yoda and his effing do-or-do-not effing bull-effing-crap effed-up wisdom."

Some of my blog followers told me to breathe. Some of them

told me to stay positive. Some told me, "Next time." Sean was not happy. I didn't mean my Yoda rampage as an assault to *his* training philosophy, but I just didn't get how it could be so black and white for him.

This question has intrigued me for years: What's the difference between a reason and an excuse? We in the health media love to do stories such as "Excuse-Proof Your Workouts." Basically, you give me an excuse, and we'll find a solution for how you can get around it. But aren't there tangible and legitimate reasons someone might not reach a goal: injury, a hectic work schedule, life situations that just get in the way? Or are these all just blabber? If you really wanted your goal, wouldn't you find a way around it?

Part of the dilemma is that there's a big disconnect between what we say and why we actually do things. "Our motivational system is a very old evolutionary system, and it does not communicate well with the rest of the brain," said Art Markman, PhD, of the University of Texas at Austin. So what we do, Markman said, is use stories to help project that system to others and help explain what we do to ourselves.

"We have access to feelings and behaviors about ourselves, and we use that information to interpret our own behaviors," Markman said. Sometimes that interpretation is very simple and easy. If you almost get hit by a bus and leap out of the way, you have a mixture of fear and relief, so you think to yourself, "Yeah, wow, I know why I'm feeling this—I almost got hit by a bus." But for a lot of things we do, it's not 100 percent clear why we're doing it. So in instances when we've failed at some goal that we stated we wanted to achieve, we tell that story. And depending on who's listening to it, you can call it a reason or an excuse. On one hand, we have privileged access to information nobody has—I know what I'm feeling, I have my own memories of what I'm seeing and hearing. On the other hand, we're just as mystified about the working of our own motivational systems that we have to guess, too.

I guess the way I settled it in my mind is that there are reasons and there are excuses, and it doesn't matter how the outside world wants to perceive them. Instead of trying to identify what's a reason and what's an excuse, it really is simply about making a choice. I chose to have (perhaps too much) Easter candy that week. I chose the race that was run on the golf course at that time of day. I made my choices, and if I wanted to reach my goal, I'd have had to make different ones.

I learned something about how to handle a perceived failure from Tony Bevis. When Tony tore his knee up on the third day of his college football career, the team doctor told him that he could do rehab and continue to play, but if he did, he might never walk right for the rest of his life. Or he could walk away.

Bevis, then 210 pounds, decided to walk—to Taco Bell.

From the moment he left the team, Tony enjoyed the college experience and started to gain more and more weight. He and his two roommates would go to Taco Bell and eat fifty tacos between them. Tony had grown up as a fan of food; his dad, as the youngest of eight children, never had a lot of food, so one of his goals was to make sure that Tony and his sister never went hungry. "I'm not blaming my parents," Tony said. "I'm the one who kept putting the fork in my mouth."

Soon he met his wife ("a really good baker, a really good cook"), and he kept gaining weight. At times he'd try to lose weight, work out a little, make excuses, and then continue to gain.

He knew it was tough walking upstairs. He knew it was tough walking a hundred feet. He knew he had to do something, but he never did. Sometimes he'd ask his wife, Sheri, to hold him accountable—to challenge him when he ordered steak and potatoes instead of healthier meals. When Sheri would say, "That's not really what we talked about eating," he'd tell her to stuff it, but a lot less politely. ("I'm surprised she's still with me," Tony said.) Other times, he'd drive up to the McDonald's drive-thru to eat a ten-piece box of McNuggets—and then have dinner when he got home. He'd open bags of chips, give a few to the kids, then blame them for eating the whole bag. "It became a sick, twisted psychological game in my head to see what I could get away with," he said.

Instead of facing the issues, he'd just buy bigger pants and bigger shorts—until he needed 5X, some fifteen years after getting hurt in college. That's when it scared him—so much so that he decided to buy a scale and see what the numbers said.

He expected to see 350.

Instead, the scale snarled back: 440.

"It was a jaw-dropping experience," he said. "I was mortified that I was that heavy. That was the moment that I decided I had to do something."

Previous attempts at weight loss had failed because he didn't see results right away. This time, Tony took a different approach. When his wife went out running with friends, he would grow tired of being left home all the time. So when she went running, he would go along—and go for a hike or walk. That's when he decided to set a goal and stay dedicated to it. He called his buddy Dave and told him he wanted to hike a 14er (a fourteen-thousand-foot peak) on an upcoming trip to Colorado.

"I think the key was that he didn't laugh at me," Tony said. "He said, 'Let's do it.'"

So Tony, who could barely hike a mile when he started, built up to hikes of ten or eleven miles. Before his trip to Colorado, he dropped forty pounds, but that still meant he was a four-hundred-pounder attempting to move up a mountain.

The day of his hike, he made it to twelve thousand feet—including a gain of two thousand feet over three hours via a winding path up the mountain—before his body crapped out on him. His muscles seized; he couldn't move. He knew if he tried to get to the top, he'd put himself in jeopardy because he still had to make it back down. Unlike others who maybe would've viewed coming up short of the goal as a loss, Tony didn't use the experience to sabotage his bigger quest. He used it as fuel.

"I wasn't disappointed," he said. "Shoot, I was a four-hundred-pound guy who got to twelve thousand feet. Not many four-hundred-pound guys can do that. And I will get back and finish the trip up that mountain."

When he got home, he started an online running program and made it down to 385 pounds before joining a local *Biggest Loser*-style competition in Kansas City. There, he changed his eating habits, started working with a trainer, and learned to make the changes he needed to lose more weight. And he learned how to deal with temptation, because he runs the kitchen of a homeless shelter. "I'm around food eight hours a day," he said. "It's hard to fix food for twenty or thirty people and still eat clean."

He's raced a 10K and a half marathon, and though he didn't win the weight-loss competition, he used it to keep himself going, to keep himself accountable—to himself and to others. He made a Top 10 list of things he wanted in his life—ride roller-coasters again, not shop in the big-and-tall stores anymore, not have to choose restaurants based on whether they have booths or tables, because booths were just too stinking uncomfortable. Now down to 330 pounds, Tony wants to make it 300, then 200. He credits the support and encouragement of his family and friends (virtual ones he's met through a Facebook group as well as live) for getting him going. He and Sheri go to friends' nearly every Friday night, and those friends decided to eat the way Tony needed to at every get-together—meaning they emphasized fruits, vegetables, and protein, and gave up the breads and potatoes. "For them to say, a hundred percent, while you're doing this, we're going to do this, that kinda blew me away, and seeing that much support from family and friends really pushed me to continue to eat well," he said.

Another factor helped him: It was having a level of accountability, but not letting setbacks (or even not accomplishing his articulated goal) derail him. It came when he called up his friend Dave to hike the 14er. It came when he committed to races, and to telling his virtual friends about them. It came when he agreed to join teammates in a weight-loss challenge. Simply the act of putting himself in the public, rather than solely setting a goal, made it work.

"Accountability is huge. I don't think I could've done it if I didn't have that accountability. Pride is a big part of that," Tony said. "For so long, I let myself go. And to see any kind of progress, you puff out your chest a little and be proud of what you've done. I just got tired of being disappointed in myself . . . If I didn't set the goal to hike the mountain, I'd probably still be sitting on the couch."

Dedication Is About What Happens Backstage, Not in the Performance

I've come to realize that dedication is the exact opposite of what we may think it is.

We like to think of dedication as emotion—as being gutsy, being loud, being grunters who push and pull and fight to reach our destination.

Real dedication is quiet.

Real dedication isn't about emotion; it's about cognition—about learning what to do and then thinking about the process to do it.

I should have known this, because I live with the person who has taught me the most about dedication: my wife, Liz, who has dedicated so much of her life since she was five to pursuing her passion for competing in equestrian events. She's gone through so many obstacles—changing disciplines after watching friends and strangers die in accidents on course, waiting out long-term injuries in her horses and not knowing what the outcome would be, pouring so much love and time into her passion for her horses and into a sport with few spectators and no mass support. She invests hours, days, months, and years into training for competitions where her rides will only last a few minutes with very little fanfare. Her rhythms go hand in hand with her horses' rhythms. How they go, she does.

I've always admired Liz's drive and passion for being so in tune with something that moves her—and she never, ever considers her hard work a sacrifice, because this *is* who she is. She is the icon of intrinsic motivation: She's not moved by ribbons or wins (though she's as competitive as they come), but by how she bonds and develops and grows *with* her horses. She's dedicated and determined not in a clench-your-teeth way, but in a love-of-the-journey way. I spent two decades knowing this, watching this, admiring this. Why did it take me so long to learn to be this way myself?

Right after my golf course 5K failure, I was pissed, but I decided to use that and learn from it. So I met with a running coach who gave me a speed program. I did workouts that I've never done before. A few months later, I signed up for another 5K, and targeted that one for my next sub-thirty attempt. I had put in the training and felt pretty good, though I didn't know if I had the wheels to drop below thirty. On race morning, I fueled up well (coffee, a bagel, and a Snickers bar) to ensure I had caloric energy to sustain me. When the gun went off, so did I. I checked my watch, and I looked to be on target. "Hold on," I kept telling myself. "Hold on." When I rounded the final turn, I turned into my kick, and my watch spat out per-mile-pace numbers that I had never seen before. Finally: 29:34. Not fast by many measures, but it was my fastest—and I had finally hit a goal I had failed to hit before. The funny thing, though, is that it wasn't about being determined *that* day. It was about staying focused on the mechanics in the days leading up to it.

I finally got Sean's point. Dedication isn't an in-the-moment "do or do not." It's about everything that leads up to that moment—to give you the ability, power, and capacity to do or do not.

10. INSPIRATION

Truth: You Will Get Most Inspired When You Try to Inspire

About halfway through the course of my second Tough Mudder, my team and I saw a big man—likely three hundred pounds—running shirtless with a Superman logo tattoo on his upper back. He was plugging through the course by himself. When he reached a wall or obstacle that he couldn't overcome alone, people around him helped him. And he kept going. We saw him a lot that day; he would pass us on certain obstacles, as it took us a while to get five of us through certain spots, but then we passed him on the run.

I wanted to say something to him. I wanted to tell him that what he was doing was an inspiration. His solo run, to me at least, was a big "screw you" to all the people who don't think big boys can bust it. But how do you say something like that with good intentions without sounding like a condescending jackass? Especially, how could I? Who was I, a man with a fair amount of fat, to say anything? No matter what comes out of your mouth, it could be interpreted as, "Way to go, fat boy! Nobody thinks you can do it." But that's why I was so inspired, because I'm sure a lot of people looked at him and thought, "WTF?" I was inspired that not only had he decided to run the course, but that he had also done so, apparently, without the safety net of a team around him. Later, I tried to track the man down, with no luck. I wanted to know why he'd done what he did, and I wanted to thank him for not giving a crap about what others thought about him—and for changing what people thought: that you don't have to be a certain size, or type, or weight to do what you want.

Just as I have a list of my favorite foods, I also have a list of all the people who have inspired me the way this guy did. Besides my wife's dedication to her horse life, I'm inspired by my twin boys, who are far superior athletes than I ever was or will be. They work hard at the gym, they hustle in the sports they play, they compete, but they never gloat or peacock around the field—and they have the kind of sportsmanship I'd want my kids to have, being humble in victory and gracious in defeat. I love Olympic athletes for their athletic prowess and their singular focus on following their dreams and perfecting their talents, especially when they know very well that they may not receive the same attention or financial reward that elite athletes in other sports do. I'm also inspired by Navy SEALs, because, well, Hell Week. I'm inspired by underdogs and behemoths. I used to be inspired by Lance Armstrong and his quote from his Nike commercial, where he said, "People ask me what I'm on. I'm on my bike six hours a day busting my ass. What are you on?" (Damn it, Lance.)

Actually, I can remember the first time I was inspired by someone using her body to push past her limits. I don't remember if I saw it unfold as it happened or some years later, but I remember the footage. It was of Julie Moss, then twenty-three, competing in the 1982 Hawaii Ironman Triathlon, which was airing on ABC's *Wide World of Sports*. She was leading the women's race, but during the run, her body shut down. She wobbled on jelly legs, she fell, she crawled. She got up. She swerved. She fell again. Just yards from the finish, she lost the lead when she was overtaken by the woman behind her. Later, Moss told the press that she spent about ten seconds feeling sorry for herself, and then she decided to get up and finish, crawling to the end. It took her a long time, she said, for her to own that moment—one that felt like failure to her but served as an inspiration for so many people to try things they didn't think they could do.

Look at what she did. Look how she got up when she was knocked down. If she can have that much heart and courage and grit, could I, just maybe, have that, too? Moss later learned how important her fight-to-the-finish was—quite possibly even more so than winning would have been.

I'm inspired by all kinds of athletes—the crazy-good ones who are at the top of their sport and the people who may not look like they belong but who give it a shot anyway. Like the guy I saw at Tough Mudder. Or the person who finishes last in a local 5K. The one racing with a prosthetic leg. The ones with not just ability but grit. They are living metaphors for what we, as people who need to lose weight, want: to just plug away and get it done. Those of us in this weight-loss fight admire the people with bodies we will never have, as well as the people in whom we see ourselves: the ones with the innards to fight on when it'd be easier to pound pancakes.

Inspiration: Fuel for Energy

Inspiration, I've always thought, is something that doesn't really need to be defined. We know it, we feel it, we use it to help take us to the next place where we want to go. I've always seen inspiration as a little more soulful than what we may label our day-to-day motivation—there's something deeper going on. So I asked researcher Art Markman what the difference was between the two. Motivation, he said, requires both a combination of a well-defined goal and the energy to pursue that goal. Inspiration is only one piece of the motivational formula—the energy part. "If you look at the field of motivational speakers, they tend to break down on one or the other side—goals versus energy. Some speakers convey to the world that you need to focus on your goal and how you can structure your life so you can achieve certain things," Markman said. "The former football coaches, the generals, and CEOs, they're all about energy." Markman was also quick to point out that energy without direction is wasted, but direction without energy is frustrating—meaning that we all need both principles in play.

"That becomes the very difficult point," he said. "When you're not seeing progress, then that's when energy starts to fade."

That's why weight-loss journeys can be so difficult and frustrating, Markman said. Because weight loss is not a linear progression—meaning that there will be many times when we don't see that progress on the outside, even if changes are being made chemically and metabolically that are good for our bodies— we assume that what we're doing is wrong, and then we bail. "Without those markers of progress, we're prone to look for other strategies that give us immediate feedback that we're doing something right," he said. "But the human motivational system doesn't have a progress bar like when you're installing a piece of software."

Even when changes are happening, if we don't see them, we abandon our plans, including what may in fact be working. Which is why the idea of inspiration—of using energy to feed our actions—needs to be part of our weight-loss formula. The dilemma, though, is that you can't simply order up inspiration in the same way you can order up a side of steamed vegetables.

In a paper in the *Journal of Personality and Social Psychology*, researchers Todd M. Thrash, PhD, and Andrew Elliot, PhD, aimed to establish inspiration as a mainstream construct in psychology. Some important characteristics of inspiration, they wrote, are this: Inspiration is evoked (rather than willed to appear, as with motivation); it involves transcendence above the ordinary; and it moves us to act on a new idea or vision (this is called approach motivation). While original meanings of inspiration involve some kind of supernatural influence (think of the Muses), they wrote, most psychologists reject that as a key component. Thrash and Elliot developed an Inspiration Scale, and found that those who scored high on it also did well in other areas of life. In a piece in *Psychology Today*, Scott Barry Kaufman, PhD, a cognitive psychologist at New York University, wrote about why inspiration matters and about some of Thrash's and Elliot's research. Kaufman made the point that recent research shows that inspiration doesn't have to be solely out of our control. He wrote, "Contrary to the view that inspiration is purely mythical or divine, I think inspiration can be thought of as an interaction between your current knowledge and the information you receive from the world."

Which begs the question: How can we, and should we, try to control it? Can we figure out ways to use inspiration to give us the energy to go through the processes that will work, rather than letting inspiration come to us the way it perhaps should, naturally and unpredictably? I read Kaufman's comment about "information you receive from the world" with the message that inspiration is really about exposing yourself to, for lack of a better term, different kind of data. The more I can see, the more I can interact with people. The more I can observe other people's lives, the more lessons I can draw from them and apply them to my own struggles. It's not about being told what to do, or of reading a plan of do-this and do-that actions and trying to follow every step perfectly. It's about creating our own stories and using other people's stories to inform our own. The missing part of the inspiration equation for many people is that, most times, we're looking to be the receiver—we're looking for that data that can help us. We want to be moved. We want that energy. We want inspiration thrust upon us. What we don't realize, perhaps, is that when we start to receive it, we begin to give it—and that's the cycle that has the *most* energy.

The Inspiration Feedback Loop

Several years ago, Kim Johnson, who admittedly has been thick and pudgy her whole life, lost fifty pounds. She did it for one reason: Her middle-school daughter was gaining weight, and she wanted to help her. She knew she would have no credibility if she herself needed to lose weight. "I knew I was not able to pass the red-face test. If I'm going to give someone advice, it's hard to do that if I can't follow it myself," she said. "I knew I needed to practice what I was getting ready to preach, so I decided to do something about it." She joined Weight Watchers and started doing some strength routines with a trainer. She lost thirty pounds quickly, stalled, but then ramped back up after she started running. (She's since run fifteen half marathons and five marathons, and gets a lot of her joy from fitness through running a lot of races of all distances.) Her mix of strength training and running has helped her maintain her weight loss.

Kim tries not to push too hard with her daughter—she doesn't want to be a drill sergeant, but she does want to model healthy behavior.

"I know she's proud of her races . . . she wears the shirts to school. I just have to be careful what we sign up for—a Did Not Finish would be devastating for her. So long as she's having fun, that's what's important to me. I want her to have good memories of fun times doing races together," Kim said.

"I know she sees my efforts, but I'm not always sure the best way to be encouraging without being overbearing—there's really a fine line there. My daughter doesn't like to train, but she loves the races. So I find races with longer time limits so we can enjoy ourselves without the pressure of a sweeper behind us. I wish I could say she's lost her weight, but she hasn't—yet. But I've planted a kernel of possibility. I can provide a model, so she will know how to do it, but she's got to find the motivation inside herself. Until then, I'll just keep running."

Kim draws a lot of her own energy from training and racing with Team Red, White & Blue, an organization that supports veterans as they transition to civilian life. Every race she goes to, she runs into people wearing their eagle emblem shirts, so she never feels alone.

When it comes to the physiology of our bodies, one of the driving forces is that of feedback loops—when one thing happens, that causes a reaction, and those two systems talk to each other. Sometimes feedback loops take place to balance out the systems in your body, and sometimes they handle a problem. When your body temperature rises, for example, your body tries to cool it down (with sweat). Or if you get stressed (wild animal bearing down on you), your body opens up your blood vessels to get blood moving so you can hightail it out of there. Our systems talk to each other chemically to keep you alive. In a way, inspiration works like a feedback loop—if we can balance receiving and giving inspiration, the giver receives and the receiver gives (much in the way that Kim wants to help her daughter).

I think that's part of the reason I appreciate the forum I have on the *Runner's World* website. One small part of me doesn't like my label as author of *The Big Guy Blog*—that I'm automatically the outcast, the frump among the fleet. More so, I love that I can write to share my experiences—some because they're funny, some because they're revealing, and some (I hope) because they may just help someone like me move from the recliner to whatever starting line they want without worrying what others think and to let them know that there *are* people who have the same struggles.

Can I tell you whether I've actually helped anyone? Of course not. I hope that I have. I hope that I can get inspiration to work two ways: that it can be taken when you see it, then passed on to someone who needs it.

Socialize Your Struggles

For so many people, living life overweight is about as isolating and as private as it gets. You're fat. You don't want to do anything. You sit inside. And your life adventures come in the form of choosing between the barbecue chips or the sour-cream-and-onion ones. The less you need to interact with others, the better—because you run few risks of having an embarrassment, an incident, a thigh-chafing so bad that you bleed through your shorts. So you sit and watch, rather than get up and do.

The explosion of social media, blogging, Instagram, and endless selfies changed that. Now we want to connect—but we can do it safely, through the computer or phone, controlling the message, and getting positive vibes (with the admitted risk of trolling, too) from people we don't even know.

For me, writing for *Runner's World* not only gave me an outlet to tell stories about the angst and obstacles of the cookie-loving set, but it also forced me to buckle down. I had struggles, but I still had to be accountable. It's a common theme for many folks who lose weight: "I started a blog, and I didn't care if only two people read it. It forced me to be accountable." And then what they found is two people grew to ten, which grew to a hundred or a thousand, or just stayed at two. They found that it wasn't about the size of the audience, but the fact that they *had* an audience. That audience interacted with them—giving advice, virtually applauding them on, maybe even giving them a kick in the butt when they felt sorry for themselves. These blog writers got the kinds of things they could have (and may have) received in person, but they felt more connected knowing they'd have to fess up to the world about their burger binge.

For so many of us, being public is the exact thing that scares the hell out of us—removing a shirt at the beach, taking up two seats on a public bus, going to the gym where people half our size can see us sweating and struggling. So we resist. But being public is also what can draw us out to utilize the help from others—a critical form of the inspirational feedback loop: telling your story, hearing the stories of others, and then both sides feeding off the created energy.

Publication includes more than just posting words and pictures. Putting yourself out there, in person, is also a form of publication, an announcement that you're willing to look like a dump truck, but you don't give a bleep anymore, because you have a bigger goal on your mind. Publication is anything that moves your journey from private to on a stage: announcing your intentions to your family, walking outside instead of on a basement treadmill, declaring your intentions to hike up a mountain to your friend, joining a weight-loss group, blogging, using the #tweetyourweight hashtag. As is the case with many folks who fight fat, I have issues about the way shorts make my butt look or how slow I must appear when I'm plodding along the highway. But at some point, when you realize that the public can help you as much as hurt you, you see that the rewards of putting yourself out there might be worth the risks.

One day, as I ran through the neighborhood on a downward swing of weight loss, a minivan pulled up alongside me. I assumed the driver wanted directions, so I took my earphones out. I slowed to a stop, and she rolled down her window.

"I have to tell you. You look amazing. I've been watching you for the last few months," she said, in a not-at-all-creepy way, "and you just look great."

I thanked her, put my hands together like I was praying, and bowed, in a not-at-all-awkward way—just wanting to give her some kind of gesture that showed how much I appreciated the ten seconds she was taking to stop and say something. I had no idea who she was—she didn't introduce herself—she'd just felt compelled to tell me that she had noticed my body had changed. Her words acted as a verbal shot of caffeine as I finished my run—high-octane cerebral fuel, the kind we all crave.

We get those spiritual jolts only if we put ourselves out there, the way Tony Bevis did. He had every reason to stay inside, try to go at it by himself. Why put yourself out there when you're four hundred-plus pounds? Why put your pride on the line? Why take any more embarrassment than you already have to in your day-to-day life? Because when we're upfront with our problem, it's no longer about hiding from the scorn; it's about using other people's energy to help power us, motivate us, move us. To do that, we have to be willing to show our bellies—sometimes literally, sometimes just symbolically—to the world.

For example, a study of about one hundred people published in the journal *Translational Behavioral Medicine* found that people who regularly used Twitter as part of a mobile-based weight-loss program lost more weight than those who didn't. Besides the influence that technology has had on self-monitoring, it also helps with another aspect of weight-loss success: support. "We've known for a while that announcing your goals to real-life friends helps, because people can encourage you and know not to sabotage you. That's an important characteristic of virtual environments as well," said Brie Turner-McGrievy, PhD, the study's lead author who studies how emerging technologies help create health behavior changes. The advantage of mobile technology over more traditional forms of support, Turner-McGrievy said, is that it allows people to get support when they need it. In past models, someone struggling might have to wait until a group session or a weekly weigh-in or until he or she got home from work to get the support—and then it might be too late. Doughnut done. "In the virtual environment," she said, "if you're at a friend's party and there's bad food, you don't know what to do, you can get that support right as you need it."

We have to accept some amount of risk if we do want to take our weight-loss quests public. My performance coach friend Doug Newburg would say that there's a big difference between the idea of playing and that of performing. When you go from playing (doing something you love) to performing (doing that thing in public), you open yourself up to both criticism and support. That's one of the ways we seek approval—and a way to keep us moving forward, thinking that someone else is watching.

If you announce that you want to complete a challenge and then fail to do so, you can feel like you're a doof—unless you're like Tony Bevis, who was able to look at the good part of not making it all the way up fourteen thousand feet, in that he reached a higher level than most men his size would have been able to. Now, if you're looking for approval and don't get it, you risk feeling disappointed, pissed. That, Newburg said, drives many people to work harder, which doesn't always translate into success. The public values the "work hard" approach, even though the smart approach may be what makes you successful. Even if you don't reach your goals, the thinking goes, you worked hard and you deserve applause for that. The real internal struggle that goes on involves finding that balance—not wanting to risk too much of ourselves in public, but still wanting to chase down what we want with our bodies. Many people have found that the blog, the on-line confessional, is the way to balance it all. (One interesting study presented to a conference of the Association for the Advancement of Artificial Intelligence by researchers at the University of Texas at Austin found that weight-loss success was significantly predicted by a greater use in the blogs of words associated with sadness, such as *cry* and ingestion-related words such as *eat*, but not as much with words about positive emotions or health. The group, using text analysis, looked at thirteen thousand entries generated by more than two hundred and fifty users.)

In a research article published in the journal *Sociology of Health & Illness*, Australian and New Zealand researchers explored the topic of the weight-loss blogosphere. They explained that the reasons people blog about weight loss fall into several categories, besides just being a way to self-report personal experiences. They also do it, first, "to offer critical commentary on fatness"; second, as a means of catharsis; and third, to engage in informal social support systems. Perhaps the way that weight-loss bloggers differ from other bloggers, the researchers wrote, is the sense of accountability they feel. They also said that blogging about weight loss presents some complex issues—namely, how bloggers choose to portray themselves (and whether those portrayals are authentic), and how much of a person's life should be public or private. Finally, the publication of someone's weight-loss goals provides a different kind of challenge. The researchers wrote, "We note a certain tension implicit in weight-loss blogs. The aspiration of the blogger is to lose weight; once that weight loss is accomplished, the journey is over, the story is finished, and the reason for the blog is realized."

Robby L. has been doing some sort of blogging since the late

1990s, but her first public venture into blogging came in 2009, when she started the blog *FatGirl vs. World*. While some people blog as a career or because they have an audience and a unique voice, Robby says she's always been a write-for-yourself kind of blogger, doing it as an exercise in self-awareness. In this blog, Robby tried to work through her weight issues and deal with the loss of her mother when she was thirteen. "I write to finally be able to put words to pain that I had been stuffing down with food for many years," she said.

At age sixteen, she was her highest weight, 240 pounds. By 2006, she had lost about 20 pounds on her own but knew she needed help to make substantive changes in her life. To lose the rest, she joined a gym and got a trainer. Soon after finding her momentum at the gym and with food logging, she was trampled at a concert and injured her back. She spent the next three months in constant pain. Doctors were unsure she'd be able to stand up straight or walk for short periods. They were reluctant to tell her she'd be able to return to the gym. Robby's orthopedist gave her the worst-case scenario: She'd come to him in a wheelchair, unable to walk at all.

"I think having to call a colleague into your restroom because you can't pull your pants up counts as a 'worst moment,'" Robby told me.

Rehab (physical therapy, epidural steroid injections) took priority over weight loss, and she stopped looking at the scale. She ate through her frustration and pain. By the time she did look, she had gained back much of the weight she'd lost before the injury.

Midway through her recovery, she had an epiphany. Instead of focusing on what she couldn't do, she decided to prove her doctors wrong by focusing on what she could do: honor every healthy day she had with proper nutrition and what she called joyful movement (a walk, swim, stretch, anything). Her inner voice told her, "Fight for yourself."

Still thirty pounds away from what she thinks her goal weight should be when we connected, Robby would rather focus on her successes than on setbacks. (At her last checkup, her doctor said she was doing better than 95 percent of his patients.) "I realize that I need to be more careful with my diet on the days when I can't exercise, and more creative with getting exercise on the days my body is giving me trouble, but the upside is that I'm very aware that the scale isn't my only measure of health," she said. "Sometimes it's just being able to put my pants on."

She opened herself up to the world with her blog, writing in the "About Me" box that she'd been overweight or obese since she was eight years old. Her first entry:

> I am a 28-year-old, size 14, 5'9", 217lb woman. I know I'm obese. I know I am fat. I also know that I'm statistically average-sized. I do not have my own gravitational pull.
>
> I do not eat Twinkies, eat fast food, or guzzle soda. I play sports. I can even run. I know what a basal metabolic rate is, and I frequent farmers markets.
>
> I have heard your putdowns. I've been on your diets. I've been the butt of many of your jokes. I have suffered your insults, both the shallow ones and the ones that cut deep to my fat-laden core.
>
> And you know what? Despite your trying to put me down at every turn, I still manage to be a happy, confident, sexy woman.

This blog is my open letter to you, World. Just know that
no matter how beaten down any entry might sound, I will
remain triumphant, positive and more than you can handle.

Sincerely,

Fatgirl_vs_World

Robby didn't expect that by being candid she'd get the response
she did: Family members and strangers were thanking her for opening up, and they encouraged her to continue to both heal and write.
That gave her the freedom (and courage) to say things she may
never have been able to in the past.

"The surprise," she said, "is finding out that John Donne is
right: No blogger is an island. We're all connected. When one of
us has a victory, we all celebrate. When one of us struggles, the
rest of us form a net. Sometimes I've been the victor; sometimes
I've needed the net."

That net is the thread that ties together inspiration—the connection between the giver and receiver of the messages. Doug
Newburg has talked to me many times about why he thinks this
is the missing piece for so many people. He told me that I found
connection in writing but had trouble finding it in my fitness pursuits. "You'd sign up for things based on the excitement and nov-
elty of new things, but because they were mostly solo endeavors,
they failed," he said. He said that through my blogs, he's seen me
grow—from initially not wanting to let people down to finding
the right coaches and partners and teammates that motivate me to
push through on difficult days. This is key, he said, because research shows that the method a trainer or a therapist may use is
less important than if the person trusts that trainer or therapist.

The same principle holds true for the people you put around you. Do you trust your circle? The problem, he said, is that our society has created an environment where we chase these moments—the bliss points, as he calls them—that are sort of like an addiction. They come and go, and like any other addiction, they can cause you to crash and burn if you don't get your fix. The more productive path, he said, is establishing those connections that allow fewer crashes (often through bringing your struggles public).

"It comes down to something I've said a lot," Doug said. "Are you chasing what you *think* you want, bliss points? Or are you doing something you actually like, a small, gentle, sustainable buzz you can count on instead of a high that quickly fades?"

Truth: It Takes Others to Do It by Yourself

After running 10-plus miles, I stood at the base of Everest. Not the 29,029-foot one in the Himalayas, but a 16-foot one in Tampa. Everest is the name of one of the signature obstacles of the Tough Mudder course—a 12-mile muddy run dotted with thirty-ish obstacles. These challenges range from the freezing (submerging oneself in a Dumpster filled with ice water of about 35 degrees and then climbing out again) to the frightening (jumping off a 15-foot platform called Walk the Plank into a pond-size body of water). The course also has 10- and 12-foot walls to climb over (with the help of your team, if necessary), and a maze of electric shocks that will zap you flat on your face as you run through. I mostly feared Everest, a quarter-pipe wall. Picture a skateboard half-pipe, cut it in half; there's a rounded portion at the bottom that juts up to perfectly vertical. Your mission: Run as fast as you can up the ramp and leap for the top, attempting to pull yourself up and over.

Many good athletes can do this all by themselves.

I cannot.

I signed up for a Tough Mudder with three of my buddies (including fitness guru Adam Bornstein and Yoda lover Sean Limon) as a way to challenge myself and face fears in a new way. Our event took place in December 2011, and I mildly freaked out in September 2011, because that's when a doctor's office visit indicated I had gained thirty-some pounds since my marathon a year earlier. I had ballooned back up to 262 pounds. That was no load I wanted to carry—or wanted my teammates to have to carry— across this course. With gravity against me, I knew Everest would prove to be my greatest nemesis. In the few months before Mudder, I trained hard and ate right, and I believe I got down to about 240 or 245. (I didn't weigh myself because I didn't want to know; had the number been greater than I suspected, it would have been a fire-tipped spear to my psyche.) On race day, though, I knew I weighed more than I wanted to.

At Everest, one of the last obstacles of the day, I watched as my buddies made it up. Adam flew up. Sean zipped up. Mike climbed up. They needed to go first to have the manpower and muscle to help me up when I approached.

By myself, with hundreds waiting to try and probably hundreds more watching along the sidelines, I waited while my teammates yelled for me to run at them.

Liz, having watched many successful and failed attempts at Everest, came over. She knew I was worried. She also had no idea how the rest of the course had gone, but she wanted me to conquer this ramp.

"You have to get your leg up. That's the key. Get one leg up," she said, meaning that when my teammates grabbed my hands, it wouldn't be enough for them just to pull my arms. I had to do some work, too, flexing my inflexible body parts and lifting my leg as close to the top of the ramp as I could. More body parts to grab would mean more chance of my not looking like a jackass fool who was too fat to finish.

So I went. After having been on the course for three hours, I ran as hard as I could, jumped up, and reached . . .

Zero contact.

I hit the ramp belly-first and slid cartoon-style down to the bottom.

As I walked back to the masses, Sean yelled, "You *are* getting up here."

All I was thinking was "How am I going to do that?"

Before the race, Sean had given me instructions: "You're getting over everything. Failure is not an option." (Yoda, again.) I tried explaining why I was concerned (as if it were not obvious). Then he said something that really hit me: "If you don't make it over something, that's not you failing. That means we failed as a team to get you over. And I'm not failing." Previously, my tendency was to tell my teammates I was sorry I was holding them back, sorry they had to lift so much weight over the wall. But on this day, I wasn't going to do that. I was going to do *it*.

When I walked back to the pack after my face-plant, I really didn't know how this would work. All my teammates were on top waiting. I let a few people go ahead of me, waiting for my turn. What if this takes me ten times, twenty times? When would it be okay to say, "Enough is enough. This body just isn't made to Spiderman up vertical walls"?

As I ran to the ramp the second time, I didn't know what to expect. I saw some Mudders reach the top and some Mudders grab hands, dangle, then fall.

I sprinted, jumped . . . and felt my two hands being snapped up like a fly in a frog's mouth. And then I dangled. Flailing. Spinning my legs as if I were on a unicycle trying to do something to power up. Nothing.

"You *are* getting up here! You *are* getting up here!" Sean yelled.

Then I remembered what Liz had told me. "You have to get your leg up."

I tried to lift my left leg, but it wasn't high enough. They couldn't reach it. I lifted again.

Nothing.

Some hip-flexor exercises would have come in handy right now, I thought.

Again.

I felt a hand get my inner thigh.

They then muscled me up. I rolled on my back at the top, smiled, yelled, and said, "I fucking love you," to the group that pulled me up.

Later I asked, "How many guys did it take to get me up?"

Adam and Sean said they didn't remember.

Mike did: "Five."

Accept Help to Get Over Walls

I loved running a Tough Mudder, not just because it wasn't a timed event so I had no pressure to meet a speed goal, but also because it was all about getting over obstacles and using a team to do so. While plenty of people can do the course on their own without a leg up or a push or pull from a teammate, many of us Mudders need the muscles and the energy from each other to get through.

Even though I slogged behind, I loved it—so much so that I did another one the next year, with a few different people (where I saw the guy with the Superman tattoo). After I did that first Mudder, I felt like it changed me. I wasn't the weight I wanted to be, but I could viscerally feel more confident, and I think that experience propelled me to lose more weight. My friend Doug Newburg suspected as much. He thinks that my experience at the wall summarized my whole journey.

"How I see you and how I suspect how you want others to see you is trying to get over that wall and you being worried about how others see you," he said. "What started as a physical challenge became an unconscious emotional challenge that you can't ignore. You were really worried about it. The challenge wasn't getting over the wall. It was committing to being part of a team. You wanted to connect with people, and that's the underlying thing in everything we do. That is the goal. This is what being human is about: connecting to other people. Your wall story is so perfect. They wouldn't have been upset if you didn't get up. They would have been disappointed *for* you, not *in* you. That's such a huge thing. Once you make that shift, the weight gets lifted."

It doesn't matter whether someone lost weight through this diet or that exercise program, or in nine months or four weeks. It doesn't matter whether someone went with 30 percent protein or with giving up all forms of carbs. It doesn't matter whether someone did it through running or weights. It doesn't matter whether someone was motivated by an embarrassing photo or a life-threatening blood pressure number. The theme that's present in anybody who's had success: strong social connections.

That comes in the form of anecdote after anecdote, as well as the harder sciences. In a study published in the journal *Obesity*, researchers looked at people who were put in teams to participate in a twelve-week weight-loss program. They found that being on a team in the weight-loss division (compared to being in a division that measured minutes of activity or pedometer steps) with more teammates was associated with greater weight loss. The caveat, of course, is that social networks can also be dangerous, too: A landmark study published in the *New England Journal of Medicine*, tracking more than twelve thousand people, found that if you have an obese spouse or friends, you're more likely to be obese, too. Specifically, having an obese friend increased the chance that you'd become obese by 57 percent, and there was a 37 percent increase if your spouse was obese—numbers that drove the conclusions that we could socially "catch" obesity in the same way that we could catch a cold. The researchers wrote that it's the social network, not the physical environment, at play, since geographic distance didn't play a role, indicating that virtual networks and relationships can have as much impact as physical ones.

For a long time, the idea of needing a social network would seem like a weakness—that you need help from others because you're not strong enough to do it on your own. "The concept of social support is a dirty word in the macho world of elite sports," said Tim Rees, PhD, the University of Exeter researcher who studies competition. That attitude has shifted. Nowadays, you can't have an athlete respond to a victory without crediting those people around him or her, but it's also a tricky area, because the research also shows that people will respond negatively if the group turns on an individual—meaning it's essential that you surround yourself with the right people. "Support is important," Rees said, "but it can be devastating if you receive the wrong kind of message."

After I completed my marathon the year before Tough Mudder and wrote a race report about the successes and obstacles I
experienced that day, readers rushed to give me praise and try to
lift me up. Except one. He came out firing—criticizing my time,
telling me I didn't deserve to have a voice on *Runner's World* because I was so damn slow. It stung for a moment, but he had every
right to weigh in, and my guess is that many silent others felt the
same way: I'm too slow to rep *Runner's World*. I put myself out
there, and he deserved a chance to criticize, especially because he
made a fair point. When he posted, my loyal followers jumped
him—one in particular, a woman who only identified herself as
"curtainlady." She had been with me during my entire journey,
commenting on my blog posts, encouraging me, telling me I was
going to do okay even when I had my doubts. Though she is much
faster than I am, I later learned that she had gone through some
similar feelings as I had—seeing herself in the mirror "with not
just a muffin top but also a muffin bottom." This had sent her into
a three-week state of crying. When my troll responded, she
jumped in because his comment set her off: "We don't want you
here. You do not belong in this place."

I was okay with him being there, but "curtainlady" didn't because she recognized the power of the social network—that the
support is what helps people. During my quest to run a sub-30
5K, I started a Facebook group called the Sub-30 Club. I wanted
it to be a place where other similar runners could hang out, ask
questions, share ideas and encouragement. I thought I would get
ten or twenty people. We're now up over a thousand. The reason
I believe that it works is because people feel comfortable asking
questions, posting about failures, confessing what they've done
wrong, admitting when they chafe, and whatever it is that's

bothering them—because it's a generally safe environment where people of similar abilities are. Many folks in the club are well faster than a sub-30, and some aren't there yet, but everyone respects the feeling of not feeling adequate enough as a runner. One of the members is "curtainlady," who I now know as Laurie Canning. And here's the thing—the thing I learned from the moment she weighed in on my Marathon Virgin experience—she gets it. Even though she's much faster than a sub-30, she makes it a point to comment on nearly everyone's questions and concerns, to cheer them on, to lift them up, to empathize with the struggles. I had to ask her why—why did she help others, why did she weigh in so much, why was she the eternal cheerleader for so many people she didn't even know?

"I've just tried to stand up for the underdog my entire life," she said. "I just try to respond to people who truly need just a little bit of something. Everybody wants to be recognized. If I can do that, great. I just try to treat people the way I would love to be treated. People just want to be seen. It is all about choosing. I choose to be positive, and I choose to lift others up in the understanding that in the process, I will also help myself."

Sign of Strength: Asking—and Receiving—Help

Dacia Root grew to 286 pounds the way many Americans do: She worked a desk job, ate standard junky fare, consumed too much, didn't have any sense of portion size, and spent a decade gaining about a dozen pounds a year until she reached 286 pounds. Oh, she noticed she was gaining weight, she hated how she looked, and she never wanted to be in public. And she had plenty of low moments—like the time when a fellow military spouse approached her at a reception and said, "Oh, great—another fat Army wife." The woman was trying to connect with another person of the same size, but the remark devastated her. Is this what people think of me? After that, she was embarrassed, thinking that people must be making fun of her because of her weight.

Dacia tried to lose weight, but when she didn't see much action in the scale, she figured her method was a failure and she just stopped trying. "You just go from one extreme to another and then drop it when it didn't work immediately," Dacia said. "I just wasn't in the right space to mentally commit to do what it really takes to lose weight." She knew that if she was going to sustain it permanently, she had to figure out a long-term strategy—nothing extreme, something that was do-able.

One day, she started to break down—crying, explaining how she hated how she looked, how miserable she was all the time. That's when she realized that she was the only person who could fix herself. "I'm the only person who can commit to this. Nobody is going to make me work out. Nobody is going to change what I eat. I have to do it myself."

Dacia started with little changes. She started a blog. She tried to go for walks. She made a commitment to cook healthier dinners. She started tracking her food. Not everything worked. She started running, for example, but she knew that it hurt too much and if she got injured, it would hurt her long-term goals. "When you run and are close to three hundred pounds, you don't know what the pain means—is it normal pain because you're obese or is your body saying you're about to rip up all your cartilage?" So she figured out what she could do activity-wise. Perhaps most important, she redefined what victory meant—and what happiness meant. That came when she decided to go into unfamiliar territory.

"I took a boxing class and survived the entire class," she said. "It was maybe the worst boxing ever, but I needed to do it to find victories in more than just my weight." That class worked for the physical reasons—it burned calories, and worked both her strength and cardiovascular systems. It also worked for other reasons—it helped with her confidence, and she fed off the energy that came from group work.

She started taking some kind of class—dance class, Pilates, anything—once a day.

"I was so nervous because I felt like I didn't belong. Food was my friend. That made me feel comfortable. But I met a wonderful group of people. They never made me feel inadequate. They never made me feel anything other than beautiful. One would say, I love when you come to class, because you have the best smile and look like you're having a wonderful time. I started to feel what they saw in me—that I'm more than just a number on a scale."

Dacia lost 130 pounds—and has maintained that loss because of the small, sustainable habits she created (smaller portion sizes, eating in moderation, commuting to work on her bike). "I found my groove by finding activities I loved and eating in a way that gave me energy," she said. Her blog helped her keep a strong network (and keep her accountable), and she said that once she learned to accept herself, that's what made her successful. "Without knowing and believing that I was worth the commitment, the effort, the blood, sweat, and tears, I would have quit," she said. While I can't say there was one thing that worked for Dacia—because there were many—I can make the argument that one of the main drivers of why she stuck to better exercise and smarter food choices is because of what she gained by the people around her. That's the part of the puzzle the diet industry generally doesn't address very well: You can give me all the nuts and bolts of losing weight, but if the social connections don't help you make the choices, then the choices are more likely to become bad ones. Dacia was right in that she knew she had to do it by herself, but I'd argue that what helped her was the power of others.

Nick Swayer remembers the turning point—when he went from a big boy to a bigger boy. He didn't make the JV basketball team in tenth grade. That's when he lost motivation to stay in shape. At around the same time, he started working in the restaurant business, and later went to culinary school—not exactly the best formula for trying to be healthy more often than not. Over the years, he tried to lose weight ten, maybe twelve, times. Every time was the same story. He'd lose ten pounds, but then he'd fizzle out and give up. He'd run, wouldn't get far, decided he was no good at it, then just quit. When he turned thirty and his daughter was almost one, Nick decided he had to change. "I just got tired of being fat," he said.

This time, he did one thing he had never done before: He asked for help. His older brother had started running a year before then and lost some weight, and his younger brother was a drill sergeant—and in great shape. Nick declared a goal (a 5K race three months out) and approached his brothers, which wasn't easy. "It was like admitting defeat—that kind of feeling—that I just can't do this without help," he says. "Maybe the pride got in the way more than anything."

Once he asked, though, everything changed. His drill-sergeant brother took him to a twenty-four-hour gym at 11:00 p.m. on New Year's Day to show him workout routines and how to use the equipment. And now, his older brother, who runs faster than he does, runs once a week with him—and will check in with him if he notices that Nick isn't logging on to record his miles. Nick is close to hitting 200 pounds and hopes to get down to the 180s, and he's run three half marathons. He credits his brothers as being the force behind his change. His younger brother knows just how to push him to the point he needs to go and then can back off, and his weekly session with his older brother benefits both of them.

"It brought us together. I think for him, it's a time to vent. In his other running group, it's not superpersonal relationships, just more of a running group," Nick said. "But for us, it's a time to vent, talk, chat, and I think it's a release for both of us. That's the one run I never skip."

Find Your Own Version of Friday Workouts

I can tell you the moment that I believe my body started to change for good: When I created Friday workouts. It began as a way for two of my friends to train together once a week to prepare for Tough Mudder, but then we started adding more people, and the Friday session just grew. For the past three years (minus a few stretches that we took off for various reasons), a group of us have met every Friday for a workout that lasts at least an hour and sometimes more. Every time, I try to create something different using the equipment I have (tires!), and the group includes men, women, sometimes kids, friends, spouses of friends, sometimes people I don't know. Sometimes, it's only three of us. Sometimes, it's ten. One Thanksgiving morning—as counterattack to the

impending potatoes—we had more than twenty adults and kids
go through a workout. Every week, we lift, we run, we play—and
it's typically my most difficult workout of the week. I would argue
it's not taxing because of any of the moves we're doing in particular. It's hard because we push ourselves more when we're in the
group than we typically would if we were alone.

It's true that what we're doing is efficient for fat loss and overall conditioning, in that we're performing strength moves to build
muscle and high-intensity intervals to burn fat—and that's likely
the reason it has worked so well. But I don't think that happens if
Tim's not there pushing me and cordially jawing at me to do better, to run faster. Or if Sean's not there telling me that yeah, sure,
if I think it's okay to take a break, then go ahead and do that while
he's running another lap. Or if anybody doesn't say, "Good work,"
at the end of a tough stretch.

Are there people who work out alone and can push themselves? Of course. I know plenty of those people.

But here's what I know about myself: I gained a truck load's
worth of weight working out on my own five days a week. Because
I didn't go hard enough, I went through the motions, rationalizing that any work was quality work. That, simply, isn't true. I
started to succeed when I took responsibility for my own actions,
and used the juju of the people around me to make better decisions about those actions.

The year after my first Tough Mudder experience, I signed up
again the following year. My friend Sean was on the team, as well
as three new people—Scott (my college buddy), Shawn (a student
of a friend who was supposed to do the event but got sick right
before it), and Christine (of Taco Bell Diet fame). Having con-
quered the course the previous year, I wasn't quite as worried

about finishing. I knew I wouldn't be able to make it across the monkey bars and would likely take another dunk into the water after slipping off (which happened), and I knew that it would probably take several times to get up Everest (which also happened). But I went into the event fairly relaxed—just trying to have fun with each mile and each obstacle.

When we hit the ten- and twelve-foot-high walls, Shawn—an ROTC beast of a man, who weighed what I did, but all in denominations of muscle—lifted me up and over them. When he helped everyone else over, he stepped back, ran toward the walls, and then heaved himself up and over.

Close to the end, we came upon an obstacle I had not seen before. And I semi-panicked.

The wall appeared to be about twenty feet high with ropes dangling in front of it. I knew I'd never be able to haul my body up a rope à la gym class, so I was convinced I couldn't do it. As we got closer, we saw that a few two-by-fours were nailed to the wall. So you would put your hands on the rope, then plant your feet on the two-by-fours to get yourself up. Without hesitation, we all started up the wall, and I felt good going up. Then I reached the top, which was a small ledge, maybe two to three feet wide with assorted wood structures on it that you had to climb over—all on a narrow ledge two stories up in the air. The other side of the wall looked exactly like it did on the way up—a rope and two-by-fours. ("Uh, where's the slide to take us down?" I wanted to say.) The rest of my team quickly rappelled down no problem. They all stood at the bottom looking up, waiting for me. I froze. I didn't trust my lack of grip strength to hold the rope, but I did trust gravity to cause me to plummet to the earth ass-first, a shattered coccyx just moments away.

When my team saw that I wasn't moving—and that there was no escape route except straight down—Shawn ran up to the wall and climbed back up it. He stood next to me on top, and instead of giving me a locker-room speech trying to fire me up, he broke down the steps. Put your right hand here, now your right foot there, left hand here . . . Within seconds, I was moving down. Moments like this are what these events are about: finding the answer. Helping others and being helped—this constant feedback loop is the driving force behind why these obstacle courses have exploded in popularity. What Shawn did also works symbolically for weight loss—he broke down the seemingly insurmountable parts into the process, he did it without judgment, and he did it because he wanted to help me succeed. He did it because he knew that I could overcome what I needed to—with regard to fear and physical ability. When I got back down, I confided in Yoda Sean— the man who had coaxed me to sign up for an Ironman that was now less than a year away—that I was this close to being in real trouble, and I had a sense of that before I started.

"I almost went around that one," I confessed.

"Oh no," he replied, "I wouldn't have let you."

Truth: There Is No Finish Line

"**D**o you have your tri suit?" Sean asked.

"No," I said.

"Why not?"

I explained to him that I was waiting to buy a triathlon suit—those skintight shorts and tops that are supposed to make you more aerodynamic and hydrodynamic, make you perform better when you swim, bike, and run in a race. Sean, who's pushed me and challenged me and helped me in several athletic endeavors, somehow convinced me to sign up for an Ironman, since he'd completed one in 2010. This race—a 2.4-mile swim, 112-mile bike ride, and 26.2-mile run—is considered one of the most taxing endurance events around. It's not for people who aren't prepared. Not for people who aren't willing to put in long hours of training. Not (usually) for people who have bodies more like Peterbilts than Porsches.

So a year before the 2013 Ironman, Sean and I volunteered at the race and then signed up the next day. While in line, I looked at all the other athletes around me. Most were lean and strong.

Most probably wanted to tell me that I was in the wrong line. *(Uh, sir, the Chinese buffet is over there.)* While there, we heard someone talking about a mantra that had helped her friend complete Ironman training. "Suck it up, Princess." It stuck, and whenever I wanted to whine or explain why I had trouble fitting a workout in, I'd hear it: "Suck it up, Princess." (Hell, they didn't even know about my women's jeans.)

Three months before the Ironman and well into my year of training, Sean and I signed up to do a very short race—as a way to get me acclimated to everything. (I had done two triathlons some ten years earlier and, unsurprisingly, finished them toward the back of the pack.) The day before we left for that race, Sean asked me if I had my tri suit. That's when I told him I wanted to wait until I'd lost a little more weight before investing in one. At this point, I had made good progress with my weight and was hovering in the 220- to 225-pound range, but was still misshapen. So my plan was to wear my XXXL cycling shorts and an XXL tank top. Not the most effective option in terms of performance, but at least they would help hide my shape from the world just a bit more than the übertight tri suits that Sean thought I should wear.

No, Sean said. This was not an option. One, I needed to practice with what I would be wearing during the big race. Two, tri suits are designed to handle the moisture from the swim better than heavily padded cycling shorts.

Whatever, I thought. *If I'm going to do this, I might as well do it right.* So I stopped at a specialty store and tried one on. When I slipped the size-XL tight shorts and top over my body, I felt as if all my fat was pressing against the synthetic walls of my apparel like thousands of soldiers breaking down a castle wall. I wanted to look strong, feel like an athlete. Instead I felt as if somebody were trying to put Saran Wrap over mashed potatoes sans bowl. But I decided to buy the suit anyway. I decided to suck it up.

When we got to the hotel the night before the race, Sean looked at me and said, "You need to buy smaller shorts." He was looking at my khaki shorts, which were dropping from my waist.

"These *are* my smaller shorts," I said. "You don't understand. I could buy a smaller size, but I wouldn't be able to fit them over my hips and butt."

"You need smaller shorts," he repeated. Sean—who has the ability to tell me how great I'm doing with my weight loss one second and say I need to push harder the next—had been thrilled with my body changes over the previous few months. He'd encouraged me, noticed when I lost some pounds, and gave me plenty of back slaps for what I had accomplished.

That's when I told him I didn't really want to wear the tri suit. "You don't understand," I said again. "This thing is so tight." (Think of a tri suit as wearing Spanx on top and bottom and nothing to cover it. Yes, I know about Spanx, but not firsthand.) If I wore the suit, I would feel all jiggly and soft, especially with all those granite-hard bodies parading around the race. I wanted to wear it performance-wise, but not persona-wise.

"Try it on," Sean insisted, "and let me see."

I got it on and looked in the mirror. I was busting out of it. Some muscle tissue was visible, I think, but it was mostly adipose tissue. All I could see were the flaws. All I wanted to do was wear my baggy gym shorts and T-shirt over it. I felt I looked okay from, well, my shoulders up and from my calves down. But everything in between felt and looked mushy.

"You look fine. You look good," Sean said. "Trust me. You look a lot better than a lot of other people out there."

On race day, I wore those baggy shorts and shirt over my tri suit while I prepped my bike and gear. Other athletes peacocked around, shirts off, tights on. They had little body fat; they had nothing to hide. When I checked in, the woman asked me what division I was in.

"Clydesdale," I said, referring to the male division of racers 220 pounds or heavier.

"Okay," she said. "I need you to step on the scale."

The numbers on the digital scale fluctuated between 215 and 225 before finally landing on 226.

"What, do you have lead in your pocket?"

One of the nicest things anyone's ever said to me. Translation: No way in hell do you look 225. Her words served as a quick boost to my mojo—and as a good lesson or two: One, we're usually hardest on ourselves than others are on us. Two, most people want to support you, even if they think your Jell-O ass could stand to get liquefied. But this woman's words wouldn't be enough: I still feared disrobing from my baggy overgarments. When that time came, I slipped them off and walked to the start area. And I felt everything I didn't want to feel: That I didn't belong. Fat. What I wouldn't do to have a beer belly rather than an apple ass.

At the ocean's edge, in the seconds before the start, I finally relaxed—and thought about how my body would perform, rather than how my body would look. So I swam, biked, and ran. I had told Sean earlier that my suit wouldn't bother me on the swim or bike (because few people would be able to see me and get a sense of my body shape), but only on the run, where I felt I'd be silently scorned by all passersby. I felt good on the first two legs, and ran slowly and smoothly on the run. I was aiming to hit a time goal and concentrating on keeping my pace to do that. After I beat my time goal by two minutes, I realized that I didn't think once about what I looked like on the run. And it hit me: "Nobody gives a crap about what I look like." How self-serving to think anybody would spend one lick of time worrying about *my* body shape. Everybody is concerned about their own races, their own goals, their own issues. I have spent all this time, an entire lifetime, worried about what others think, and the truth is that they don't think a damn thing. Nor should they. I'm the only one who cares about what I look like. I think everyone is looking, but nobody is.

Coming to Grips with Your Body

In one post, Robby L. who writes the blog *FatGirl vs. World*, gave her readers a challenge based on the quote from philosopher Sri Nisargadatta Maharaj, "Make love of yourself perfect." The challenge she suggested:

- Every day have some naked time (it doesn't matter how long). Be completely naked, no cheating.
- Place yourself in front of a full-length mirror and find a way to look at yourself compassionately and lovingly *as you are right now* (i.e., do not envision how you want to look).
- If you find this hard, put your hand over your heart and softly say, "I am here . . . I am here."
- Remain in front of the mirror until your heart rate is regular, you've stopped giggling, there's no anxiety about the person looking back at you, and until you start seeing what is perfect over what might be imperfect.

- And if you can do it for only a limited time (such as if you're a parent, or live with other people), make sure when you do this that you're not distracted. Be present and in the moment.

Of all the challenges that she asks her readers to do, this was the one she had to revise, because it was *too* hard for her followers. "I think some people had panic attacks," she told me. "Some people were able to do the challenge, finding new ways to love and connect with their body. Other people were dependent on outside factors. Did they go to the gym? Did their clothes fit right that day? Were they on point with eating? Some people gave up after too many tears, considering it an impossible task." The next month, Robby revisited the challenge, but made it less demanding: Could you simply avoid bullying yourself in front of a mirror?

"Ask people to run hundreds of miles and they'll do it. Ask them to not scrutinize their bodies for imperfections, and they just can't. Ask someone to feel worthy of their own body, and it's like you've asked them to scale Everest," Robby said. "Society has taught us to be self-effacing and humble so as to not outshine others. The result is that we're all walking around on eggshells, not just around others, but also around ourselves. I say, be brilliant. Be strong. Be the protagonist of your own story."

Robby said that she realized it's not about being Clark Kent (relatable and human) or Superman (strong and nearly impenetrable); the two can coexist. "Superman lends strength to Clark Kent, and Clark Kent lends humanity and vulnerability to Superman," she said. While admittedly not perfect when it comes to self-love, she said she got closer to it first by allowing herself her blogger persona "FatGirl" (a personification of the best qualities she saw in herself) to have a voice. That left Robby (the person behind the blog) believing in herself as her own superhero. She said that FatGirl is "unapologetic about loving and caring for herself. She is unafraid to fail and pick herself up again." Most important, she says, FatGirl "taught me how to be kind to and patient with the one doing all of the hard work: Robby."

I found her point one of the most profound ones I'd come across, because it lies at the root of what so many of us struggle with when it comes to weight loss. How do you tell yourself to accept your body when your body is not acceptable?

If you accept your body for its imperfections, does that mean you then allow yourself to become complacent to the extent that you no longer have to strive for your goals of better health and a fitter body? That's where I've struggled: Does accepting my body mean accepting complacency? (Robby says the answer is no: If you accept your body as it is, that allows you to have more reasonable goals, ones that are more sustainable over the long run.) For so long, I didn't know how to hold so-called self-love in one hand and goal striving in the other. For some, growing up in destructive and abusive environments led to embodying feelings of unworthiness. Others spent so much time unsatisfied with their bodies that no mirror exercise is going to erase decades of self-loathing. But if somehow we can transition from beating ourselves up to bringing ourselves up, it can help us achieve our goals.

"People really believe they need to be self-critical to motivate themselves," said Kristin Neff, PhD, an associate professor in educational psychology at the University of Texas at Austin. "But the research strongly supports that self-compassion is more motivating than being self-critical." Neff said that people often confuse self-compassion with self-pity and self-indulgence. In a culture where we strive to be the best, where we're very competitive, where we want to be better and do better, we have a desire to excel, and we see ourselves as a flawed human if we—*gasp!*—use kindness.

In one study published in the *Journal of Social and Clinical Psychology*, researchers wanted to measure the role of self-compassion in eating. The theory goes something like this: If people use emotional eating as a coping mechanism for stress and unhealthy attitudes toward themselves, what would happen if the opposite attitudes were in play? It's the classic dieting dilemma: Those with an unhealthy diet tend to have lower perceptions of their own body image. The study's researchers, Claire E. Adams, PhD, and Mark R. Leary, PhD, wrote, "If negative self-thoughts and feelings play a role in disinhibited eating after diet-breaking, then one way to reduce these reactions might be to prevent negative self-evaluation after an unhealthy eating episode." In the small study, women were given doughnuts—chosen specifically because it's a food that is considered forbidden on most rigid diets. (They were given a choice of either glazed or chocolate glazed, in case you're interested.) At one point in the study, the women viewed a video about rain forests while having access to food to eat. At another point in the study, a researcher interrupted the video and interjected with this "self-compassion manipulation":

> You might wonder why we picked doughnuts to use in the study. It's because people sometimes eat unhealthy, sweet foods while they watch TV. We thought it would be more like the "real world" to have people eat a dessert or junk

food. But several people have told me that they feel bad about eating doughnuts in this study, so I hope you won't be hard on yourself. Everyone eats unhealthily sometimes, and everyone in this study eats this stuff, so I don't think there's any reason to feel really bad about it. This little amount of food doesn't really matter anyway.

Through a follow-up questionnaire, researchers found that those who had doughnuts and heard the self-compassion instructions ate less than those who did not have them—the conclusion being that self-compassion can help dieters who feel guilty about eating forbidden foods. The researchers said that these people may be more successful at regulating their eating because they're less motivated to eat in order to cope with negative feelings.

The tough part for so many of us is that this self-compassion doesn't feel tangible the way that calorie counting or twenty minutes of exercise does, so we're skeptical we can easily do anything about how we treat ourselves. Neff told me that self-compassion can indeed be learned, in the same way that proper nutrition and smart exercise can be. One way, she said, is to use words with yourself that you would use with a friend. While you may beat yourself up for eating fourteen Taco Supremes, you'd tell a friend on a diet that it's no big deal, move on, and eat better tomorrow. Another way, Neff said, is through physical touch. This helps the body calm down and relax, and it really facilitates your changing your language with yourself. Most of these processes work the same way, by reducing heart rate and levels of the stress hormone cortisol, so they have a soothing kind of effect.

This isn't just make-yourself-feel-good in a *Saturday Night Live* skit kind of way. There are chemical responses at work here. Neff once wrote a piece explaining that self-compassion taps into the "mammalian care-giving system" through the release of oxytocin, the bonding chemical that makes us feel trust, calmness, and connectedness to a bigger community. She concluded that self-compassion may be a powerful trigger for the release of oxytocin.

While there may be genetic differences between people's levels of self-compassion, environment plays a role, too. If you grew up in a home with a lot of conflict, you're more likely to have lower levels of self-compassion. All the research, Neff said, points to the fact that self-compassionate people are more likely to take responsibility, more likely to apologize to others, and more likely to experience guilt than shame. (Shame is defined as "I am bad," while guilt is defined as "I did something bad," and is therefore more easily fixed.)

Neff told me that the reason people fear this idea is that they equate self-compassion with weakness, but people need to know just what self-compassion is. It's not narcissism, but rather permission to treat yourself decently. Just that simple acknowledgment can change your attitude—and your behaviors. In fact, the research points to the fact that self-compassionate people set high standards and goals; they just don't beat themselves up as much when they don't reach them. This reminded me of Tony Bevis's success on the mountain. He didn't make it to the point he wanted to, but he made it farther than he may once have been able to. "It turns people's lives around," Neff said of self-compassion. "It really is quite amazing." If you can accept the fact that you're not perfect, that can be a motivational force for change. "It gives you the emotional resources to do your best," she said, "but that doesn't mean you have to be perfect."

Ask What Really Matters

The ending to my story, if we want to gift wrap it, is supposed to look like this: After decades of self-blabbering and self-blubbering and five-gallon drums of peanut butter, I hover around my goal weight. My size shrank, and so did my pants. Victory! That's the goal, right? Get to the number on the scale, game over. Then get your butt into maintenance mode and live happily ever after eating celery sticks and bean sprouts. It doesn't work that way; our endings aren't that tidy. Even more important, I've learned that maybe there are no endings.

Lately I've done some growing along with my shrinking. I did reach a weight that I'm comfortable with—around two hundred pounds—and I can tell you that I'm in the best shape I've ever been in. But I'm not anywhere near where I could be. I still have a way to go. I still could be smaller and stronger. I still play big-butt defense, and I still have these pesky hips that make pants fitting less than ideal. For the better part of a year, I've had one big question looming: Can a guy who has lived his life as a fat ass drag that same planetarium-size butt over the course of an Ironman?

Sometime before the race—before I put a judgment on myself for finishing or failing—I learned that body satisfaction can't be about my weight, or even about what happens on race day. Because no matter what happens, there will be a next step, a next challenge, a next temptation, a next something that will either propel me forward or move me back. In a way, it doesn't matter which direction the little things move me, because I feel I've finally figured it out.

I can tell you the moment when I felt a shift in the way I thought and felt.

Given my lack of balance and overall athletic ineptitude, it's likely no surprise that the two times I tried surfing, I spent more time eating foam than riding waves. The first time I tried, I was in college. One of my very best friends, Mark—a friend who once walked slowly down a mountain behind me when my boots fell apart midhike—spent much of his youth on the water. I loved his stories about waves. He told me about how he'd spend hours out there, paddling and riding, paddling and riding—and then was able to eat two dinners because he had built such an appetite. (This was also appealing.) When writing about his affection for the water, Mark described a time when a wave pounded him to the ocean floor. He felt "like a bug pinned in a display case." (This was not appealing.)

I wanted to feel what he felt. The only problem is that it took a deft mix of coordination, balance, strength, guts, and technique. When we went into the Atlantic that day, I spent maybe an hour trying to surf, and didn't even come close to getting up on the board. In fact, I spent more time trying to get the dried board wax out of my chest hair than I did in the ocean.

The second time I tried was only a few years ago. My boys had wanted to learn to surf, and I wanted to try again. So we all signed up for a lesson, in the Outer Banks of North Carolina. Small summer waves and laid-back surfer dude instructors, I figured, would make a good combination. We did about a twenty-second tutorial on the beach—"This is how you pop up"—and I knew deep down that I didn't have a shot at lumbering my body from horizontal to vertical in one fluid motion.

Once in the water, my boys made it up after one or two tries, and they spent the next two hours riding. I spent the same amount of time toppling over like a 250-pound bowling pin. I came close a few times.

"Waves were too small, man," one of the instructors said, explaining that it was easier for kids because not only are they nimbler, but they don't need much of a wave to push them along.

Waves were too small. I translated that to *Body is too big.*

I wanted to share the moment with my boys, but I left feeling okay—I had fun in the water, and I gave it a shot. My failure still loomed inside me: I wanted to ride, not just for the ride itself, but because I was tired of my body holding me back from doing things I wanted to do.

So I tried again.

A few summers ago, Liz and I took our boys to Hawaii for vacation. Earlier that year, I declared on my blog that I wanted to finally follow through and ride a wave, preferably on my feet. So the three of us signed up for a group lesson with Maui Wave Riders. When we greeted our instructor, Kelson Kihe, he set us up with our equipment, asked about our histories, and told us a bit about what we'd be doing. My boys didn't need a lesson, so they would spend the two hours learning how to do tricks such as surfing backward and other advanced moves. He looked at my size—I'd say I was around an unsurfer-like 230 pounds at the time—and said in a very Hawaiian-friendly kind of way, "You may need the granddaddy board."

He paused.

"Or maybe the great-granddaddy."

In the past, I might have been offended. That day, I didn't care. I wanted to surf, and Kihe gave me every possible chance of making it happen. After another quick on-land lesson, in which he showed us the proper way to pop up, we hit the water.

First wave: Made it to my knees. Then fell into the water.

Second wave: My feet touched the board for an instant. Then fell into the water.

Before my third wave, Kihe talked to me. He told me how to adjust my pop-up. He told me where I needed to get my eyes, he told me to break down the steps into smaller pieces, rather than try to do it all at once. With these long, small waves, I had plenty of time to make it up.

He told me I was going to do it.

I said the same. I had no excuses—a beautiful day with my family, an aircraft carrier for a board, and a Hawaiian surf teacher who looked like a football player, so he knew what it took for big boys to get up.

On that wave, he yelled, "Paddle, paddle, paddle . . . Now UP!"

In what felt like thirty seconds but was probably only three, I made it from horizontal to vertical. Eyes up, knees bent, trying to center my shaking body. I rode that wave into shore and then raised my hands in victory.

At that moment, it all made sense. I didn't need to get my body to the point where I looked good in a bathing suit or reached some number, I needed to get it to the point where I could do things I wanted. It wasn't about perfection, but about experiences. So many things worked: Kihe was able to unlock the strategies for me to work past my previous frustrations (a bigger board and the body techniques that could help me get up); I was inspired by the beauty of my surrounding and the skills of my sons; I set and announced a goal and followed through on it; I didn't try to muscle up with unabashed willpower, but instead used the smarts of others to help me reach my goal. It was all the things that worked in that one moment that could work in anyone's quest to lose weight—and reach bodily satisfaction.

Most of all, of course, what worked is that I felt connected to the people around me. When I rode that first wave, I could see Liz give me a thumbs-up from shore, and the straightforward "good job" from both of my boys were two of the greatest words I'd ever heard. After that first ride, I didn't worry about my weight or how nasty my tight water shirt was going to look on my body in the pictures that were being taken by the surf shop photographer; I just paddled back to the small breaks. And I rode another wave. And another, and another, and another.

Victory Comes in Many Forms

The night before Sean and I left for the Ironman, our families got together for dinner at our house. I had spent nine months of very consistent (and long) training—swimming, biking, running. I had put in the miles and the hours, and I knew I'd done all I could to make it, though I also knew that my paces were such that I probably would be coming close to the seventeen-hour time limit. Start at 7:00 a.m., finish by midnight. One second late and you're labeled with a "Did Not Finish." I did not want a DNF.

Liz made steak, rice, and vegetables. She wanted to send us off well fed with Sean's family and our friends Tim and Bridget—especially because she and my boys wouldn't be going to the race. This had been the source of some contention. My boys had an out-of-area lacrosse tournament four hours from my house, and my race was four hours in the other direction. I wanted them to play their game while I played mine. Liz insisted that they should all be at my race. I tried telling them over and over that this was what they loved doing, and I wanted them to go and for Liz to be there with them. She had supported me at my marathon and my Tough Mudder, and I felt selfish having my family there while I tried another crazy goal. My quest was a big challenge, yes, but it was also still a hobby. So I pushed them away.

I never told them the reason I insisted that they not come see me.

I did not want them to see me DNF. I didn't want them to have to figure out what to say to me if I got pulled off the course for being too slow, or cramping up, or being the first Ironman competitor to pull over midcourse and order a number 6 at the drive-thru. I didn't want them to see me come up short with something I had worked toward for the better part of the year. I didn't want them to see me fail. I didn't want them to see me in the same way I felt all my school peers used to see me: as the dumpy boy who could not compete.

That night at dinner, Liz pulled up a video that was made by Tim and members of the Sub-30 Club I started on Facebook. Tim included clips from *Rocky* and *Hoosiers* and *Miracle*—and all the great underdog movie scenes he could, and he edited a video of dozens of members telling me that I could do it, that they believed in me, and that if things got bad, I should just "Suck it up, Princess." In the video, they told me over and over that they had my back.

On the days before the race, Sean noticed I was surprisingly calm. And I was. I did what I could do training-wise—"The hay was in the barn," as my friend Bill told me—and all that was left was to go to the athlete dinner. There, while most people strutted around wearing shirts boasting of past races, I wore a shirt with a picture of a cartoon runner chasing a piece of bacon.

On race morning, after a 3:30 a.m. wake-up, Sean and I downed our megacalorie breakfasts—one of the advantages of training so much is that you do get to eat a lot—and we made our final preparations. On my arm, I wrote in marker three things: a doodle of hay being in the barn, *SIUP* (for Suck it Up, Princess), and *EAT*. *EAT* was a reminder that I needed to stay fueled throughout the day, yes, but I wrote it because E-A-T were the first initials of my wife and two sons. They were the real fuel.

Five minutes before the gun sounded and before he left me to run his race, Sean grabbed my head and we looked at each other goggle-to-goggle. He instructed, "You got this. You will be an Ironman. Eye of the tiger, eye of the tiger."

One last song—"Can't Hold Us," by Macklemore—played and then three thousand-some racers darted into the Gulf of Mexico, with 140.6 miles ahead of them. Despite being kicked in the gut, my swim went well; I got out of the water at a time closer to my ideal time than to my expected time. When I got on the bike, I vowed to stay steady and not panic when I hit hills and wind. It turned out that the wind smacked me harder than I had hoped, and harder than I trained for, but I tried to stick to my plan and trust in my training. I wanted to be off the bike by 4:00 p.m. at the very latest, which would give me eight hours to cover the marathon distance. I got behind, went slower than I wanted, and didn't get onto the run until 4:45 p.m. That was still plenty of time, I knew, but not by much. (Remember, my only marathon was six-plus hours—and that was without 112 miles of biking and 2.4 miles of swimming before it.)

My plan was to run two minutes and walk one. Repeat, repeat,

repeat. The bike took more out of me than I thought it would, and I developed a county-size blister on the ball of my left foot from pedaling. I did the first mile running and walking, but my entire upper body cramped every time I started and stopped running. So I had to adjust: I would walk as fast as I could until mile five, then reevaluate. "Just stay on track," I told myself. Only mission: finish before midnight.

After mile five, I did what I could running-wise—and the only rhythm I found was telling myself to run one hundred steps whenever I could and just walk as fast as I could until I was ready to run again.

My calculations kept telling me that I was going to be okay, but then I heard something on course that made me panic. A runner was about ten minutes ahead of me (we crossed paths as the course doubled back) when a woman he knew rushed up to him because he was being projected to finish at 11:50 p.m. The race used online course trackers to give viewers updates as to their completed times at certain points, as well as projected finishing times. She yelled, a bit urgently, in his ear, "You have to move and you have to focus!"

When I heard that his projected time was 11:50 and I was ten minutes behind him, I freaked that I might not be on track to make it. The next mile was my fastest mile of the run.

Then I remembered what Sean kept telling: Stay in your bubble, don't worry about other people's races, just do what you need to do. So I looked at my watch and told myself I was still okay pace-wise. The reason this fella was projecting to be at 11:50, even though he was ahead of me, was probably because his pace kept slowing down, and they were calculating additional slowdowns. So I kept on.

Not until I reached mile twenty-four at a little after 11:00 p.m. did I know that I would make it. I had two miles left and less than an hour to do so. I tried to soak up the last few miles. People clapped. Athletes who'd finished hours before me, already showered and fed and well napped, leaned over onto the course to cheer. "You got it now," they yelled as the back-of-the-packers slugged away, trying to chase the dream. I thought about Sean and all his help that had gotten me to this point. I thought about friends who had encouraged me. I thought about my Sub-30 Club and the video they'd all made for me. (Turns out folks had made more than six hundred comments to a status update on that Facebook page as they tracked my times during the race.) And I thought about Liz and my boys, who had supported me for the entire year and who must have had an equal mix of pride and relief when it was all over. (Liz later told me that she had to go into the hotel bathroom and cry because it was unclear as to whether I'd make it before midnight, according to the real-time tracker she was following.) The power of all those people propelled me to the end.

In the last half mile, my pace quickened. The crowds were loud. I high-fived as many people as I could, screaming, "That's what I'm talking about!" over and over and over. And then a few steps from the finish line, right as I stumbled and almost took a face-plant, I heard my name, "Ted Spiker . . . You are an Ironman."

The clock read 16:39.53—just over 20 minutes to spare.

I did not "Did Not Finish."

At the end, I saw Sean, who had had his own struggles in the race (but having crushed it a few years earlier, he had said all along he was more concerned about my race than his). And I know *he* was proud and relieved—namely because he would have been the one to have to deal with me if I hadn't made it. He handed me my phone, which had messages from Liz, my boys, family, and friends, congratulating me, mostly in the form of an all-caps "YOU ARE AN IRONMAN."

Sean had taken his gear back to our room, but he was still hanging on to his bike. While searching for my postrace pizza (of which I had four slices), I asked him why he didn't take his bike back.

If it got too close to midnight without my being in sight, he said, he had planned to ride down the course, find me, and will me to the line before the midnight deadline. That gesture was *it*. Even though he had just finished an Ironman of his own, he wanted to do whatever he could within the rules to push me to a place I never dreamed I could go.

I finished the Ironman, but the race taught me that I'll never be finished. The journey, the connections, the little moments, the inside jokes, the small steps, the experience, the good-spirited "Suck it up, Princess" messages from friends, the willingness of my speedier training buddy to find my slagging butt on course if he needed to, the symbolism of climbing my own personal walls, the encouragement from my family and friends—those matter more than the time on a race clock, the number on a scale, the size of my pants, the score I got on the Presidential Fitness Test.

Afterward, I too felt proud and relieved, and enjoyed the congratulations notes I received. When I wrote my race report for my blog, someone posted a link to it on Facebook, and many congratulatory comments followed.

One reply stood out, not so much for the words ("I'm proud of you"), but for who said them: my middle-school gym teacher.

Acknowledgments

This book is one I have thought about in some shape or form for most of my pants-stretching adult life. I had always envisioned one place where I could tie together my story, the stories of others, and some of the science of weight loss to present what I hope evolved into a hybrid of information and inspiration about the nuances of weight-gain frustration and weight-loss success. I appreciate all those people who shared with me their stories, insights, and wisdom about the subject. Many of them are cited throughout the book, and while some are not, I thank them all for the time they spent to help answer my questions.

Thank you to my agent, David Black, who believed that my voice would resonate with readers and who pushed me throughout the proposal process to frame my message in a way that would work best. I appreciate his belief in my story, especially when dealing with a subject tackled as often as weight loss is. Thanks also to Sarah Smith of the David Black Agency for additional help throughout.

No book comes together without work from a behind-the-scenes team. While I'm fortunate to have my name on the front, the contributions of the good people at Hudson Street Press and Penguin have been extraordinary. Thank you especially to Caroline Sutton, the editor in chief of Hudson Street Press. Her wisdom and edits—about the big picture and lots of little ones—were always spot-on and changed this book for the better more times than I can count. I only wish that every writer could have an editor like her. Other people there who deserve my thanks include Christina Rodriguez, Brittney Ross, Courtney Nobile, John Fagan, Ashley Pattison McClay, Susan Schwartz, Norina Frabotta, Lavina Lee, Jenna Dolan, Jaya Miceli, and Eve Kirch. I also had some help when it came to very early research of what I wanted to cover in this book and some last-minute research I needed to solidify in some areas. Thanks to my former University of Florida students Naomi Piercey and Amelia Harnish for that assistance. And thanks to my friend Tim Sorel for all he did to help me pull together my video trailer for the book.

My past and present colleagues at the University of Florida have helped me not only be a better teacher, but also a better thinker and, I hope, a better writer. Thank you for your support—whether direct or indirect—of my work. I'd also like to thank my students at UF (and previously at Delaware and Lehigh), many of whom are incredible inspirations. I'm so thankful for our time in the classroom, and especially for those people who aren't just former students, but people I now consider friends. I learned I wanted to be a professor when I was an undergrad at the University of Delaware, and I especially thank Dennis Jackson and Bill Fleischman for their influence there and after I graduated. At the Columbia University Graduate School of Journalism, Sandy Padwe and Judith Crist pushed and challenged me—and made me understand what high expectations mean.

I got my first real taste of health and fitness writing from my time working as an editor at *Men's Health*, and I know that any success I may have in this business is because I had the opportunity to work with such smart and creative people there. They taught me about how to balance solid research with an engaging voice. I also have to thank the great people at *Runner's World* for welcoming me into the fold of running voices. I know I'm a nontraditional runner, and while sometimes that makes me feel out of sorts, I appreciate that they've allowed me to represent that part of the running community. Much thanks to Mark Remy, who initially brought me on as the Marathon Virgin; Chris Kraft, who now oversees Runnersworld.com, where my *Big Guy Blog* lives; David Willey, the editor in chief of *Runner's World*; and all of the editors I get to work with there. One of the benefits that came from my blog at *Runner's World* was the development of the Sub-30 Club I started to give runners like me a common place to connect. Their support, laughs, and willingness to help others are unmatched. I will never forget what they (especially Lonnie, Laurie, and Christine) did for me to help get me through my Ironman. While many people I have talked to throughout my career have deeply influenced my thoughts on health and fitness, I have to thank the following people especially: Doug Newburg, for making me see the world (and my body) in different ways than anybody else has; Jeff Plasschaert, who always treated me like an athlete, even if I felt far from one; and Adam Bornstein, whose knowledge and fire about the subject always made me want to be better.

While this is my first solo book, it isn't the first book I've worked on. First, I have to thank Dave Zinczenko for giving me my start in books. It was a pleasure to work with one of the savviest minds in the industry. He's been at the helm of many projects that have changed the lives of millions, and I appreciate the chance to have worked with him on some of them. I also spent many years working closely with Dr. Mehmet Oz and Dr. Michael Roizen, as well as a slew of others on the YOU: The Owner's Manual series of books. I cannot begin to thank Mehmet and Mike for how they've influenced my career. To be able to work so closely with two of the smartest and most inspiring people in the health field has been an honor. I learned so much from the entire experience of collaborating on the YOU books, and I am very proud to be part of that team. Thank you for an opportunity that turned into a springboard of lifelong learning.

I hope that one of my main messages that comes through in this book is the power of connections in helping people achieve their goals. I've been fortunate to have many such personal connections, especially as they relate to the pursuit of athletic or weight-loss goals. They include: my old-man hoops crew; my Friday workout buddies; members of both my Tough Mudder teams; my college friends Mark Nardone and Scott Tarpley, who I've shared many adventures with; Bill Stump, who I've always appreciated because he knows the absolute right mix of pushing and supporting; Tim Sorel, who would run right on your heels—both literally and symbolically—every single step to help you go a little faster; and Sean Limon, who flat-out Yoda'd me to reach goals I never dreamed I could.

I do wish that my father would have been alive to see his children grow up. Though he died when I was too young to remember him, I hope that I have been able to carry on some of his best traits. Thank you to my mother, Faith, for wanting nothing more than to see her three children succeed and for supporting us in our endeavors, even when she did worry about some of them. Thanks also to my whole family for their interest and encouragement of my pursuits: my sisters, Kathy and Kim, and their families; my in-laws, Karen and John, and the entire side of the Kane family; Axel and Debra and their families; my aunt Betty; and so many other family friends who've been there for me throughout.

I wish I had adequate words to thank my wife, Liz, and my sons, Alex and Thad, and to tell them what they have meant to me. To Liz, thank you for your love, for making me laugh, and for teaching me about passion, about dedication, about authenticity. And thank you for all of the influence you had over the creation of this book. Thank you, simply, for being a wonderful wife. Alex and Thad, as you grow up to be the fine young men that you already are, thank you for giving me so much to be proud of in all areas of life—your talents, your compassion, your sportsmanship. Carry these things no matter where you go and what you do. I love you all very much.